María del Pilar Díaz Martínez

Physiotherapeutic treatment by dry needling

María del Pilar Díaz Martínez

Physiotherapeutic treatment by dry needling

Upper limb

ScienciaScripts

Cover image: www.ingimage.com

This book is a translation from the original published under ISBN 978-613-9-43417-6.

Publisher:
Sciencia Scripts
is a trademark of
Dodo Books Indian Ocean Ltd. and OmniScriptum S.R.L publishing group

120 High Road, East Finchley, London, N2 9ED, United Kingdom
Str. Armeneasca 28/1, office 1, Chisinau MD-2012, Republic of Moldova, Europe
Printed at: see last page
ISBN: 978-620-8-28556-2

INDEX

TABLE OF CONTENTS....................1

1. FUNDAMENTALS OF DRY NEEDLING (PS)....................2

2. DRY NEEDLING TECHNIQUES....................20

3. PS OF NON-MYOFASCIAL TRIGGER POINTS (NMTP)....................32

4. CLASSIFICATION AND PS IN THE PGM OF THE DIFFERENT MUSCULATURE........36

BIBLIOGRAPHICAL REFERENCES....................115

1. BASICS OF DRY NEEDLING (PS).

1.1. Anatomical considerations for PS.

Dry needling involves certain risks to various anatomical structures, such as organs, nerves and blood vessels. Therefore, it is essential that practitioners have a solid anatomical knowledge, both theoretical and practical, to minimize complications (1, 2, 3, 4).

- Pleura and lungs: Pneumothorax is a serious, although rare, complication of PS. It can be avoided if the physiotherapist applies anatomical knowledge correctly. It is essential to avoid directing the needle into the lungs or intercostal space. Use the pincer palpation technique to puncture muscles such as the trapezius, pectoralis and latissimus dorsi, or direct the needle into bony structures, such as ribs or scapula, to prevent access to the pleura.
- Blood vessels: It is crucial to identify and avoid blood vessels. Knowledge of vascular anatomy allows the clinician to avoid puncturing superficial veins by inspection and palpation of arteries by pulse. Apply pressure to ensure hemostasis after needle withdrawal, especially in patients with thrombocytopenia.
- Nerves: Needle insertion near nerves requires caution to avoid injury. If the patient experiences sharp, electric pain, the needle may have touched a nerve. The area near the spinal cord and the suboccipital area should be avoided due to the risks of affecting the brainstem.
- Organs: The physical therapist should be aware of the location of internal organs to avoid punctures. For example, there is a risk when puncturing the psoas major or quadratus lumborum muscles due to the proximity to the kidney, or when approaching the abdominal muscles near the peritoneal organs.
- Joints: It is important to avoid puncturing joints, joint capsules or bursae, as it can lead to infections in these sensitive structures.
- Prostheses and implanted devices: Avoid puncturing near prostheses (limbs, internal and external fixations) or implanted devices (pacemakers, breast or buttock implants, etc.) to prevent infection and damage to the devices.
- Pathological areas: It is also crucial to avoid areas affected by acute inflammations, infections, varicose veins, cysts, tumors or skin lesions to avoid further complications.

With this knowledge, clinicians can minimize the risks associated with PS by applying appropriate techniques and taking the necessary precautions.

1.2. Therapeutic effectiveness and indications in dry needling.

1.2.1. Therapeutic effectiveness.

The key to effective dry needling (DP) is accurate diagnosis of myofascial trigger points (MTrPs) and myofascial pain syndrome (MPS). Without proper diagnosis, SP can be unsafe and generate questionable results.

The first clinical trial in which SP was used to treat musculoskeletal pain was in 1941, although the term "dry needling" was not used until 1947. This study compared three groups of patients with low back pain, one group received novocaine, another patient received saline and the last group received only the puncture. Surprisingly, the results were similar in all groups, suggesting that the needle itself had a therapeutic effect. Since then, multiple studies have demonstrated the effectiveness of PS, similar to that of anesthetic infiltrations. Subsequent research, such as that of Hong in 1994, confirmed that both PS and lidocaine infiltration are effective when eliciting local twitch responses (REL), although PS eliciting REL is more effective than infiltration without REL (5).

Despite the clinical evidence in favor of PS for numerous conditions, such as myofascial pain, neck and low back pain, headaches, migraines and more, more research is needed. Systematic reviews indicate that PS is effective, but superiority to placebo has not yet been demonstrated, posing challenges in the design of double-blind, controlled studies. Although placebo needles exist, they can generate physiological stimulation that complicates assessment of their true placebo effect. In an effort to address these challenges, some recent studies have applied treatments under anesthesia to ensure adequate masking, with promising results. Current evidence increasingly supports the use of PS, especially for immediate pain relief in patients with MDS, although further research is recommended (6, 7, 8).

1.2.2. Indications for dry needling.

Indications for dry needling (DP) refer to conditions in which this technique has been shown to be effective or its use is suggested. Among the main indications are (6, 7, 8):

- Myofascial pain: Pain caused by the presence of myofascial trigger points (MTrPs) in muscles.
- Shoulder pain: Including pain in hemiparesis, chronic subacromial syndrome (impingement), and adhesive capsulitis.
- Chronic lumbar and cervical pain: Associated with cervical or lumbar radiculopathies and whiplash syndrome.
- Headaches and migraines: For the treatment of tension headaches and chronic migraines.
- Post-surgical pain: In cases of chronic postoperative pain in the thorax or knees.
- Carpal tunnel syndrome and other nerve entrapments.
- Tendinopathies: Pain caused by inflammation or degeneration of tendons.
- Plantar fasciitis: Chronic pain in the sole of the foot.
- Chronic pelvic pain: Associated with muscular conditions.
- Piriformis syndrome and sciatica: radiating pain in the leg.
- Muscle spasticity: In patients with cerebral palsy or incomplete spinal cord injury.
- Phantom limb pain: In post-amputation patients.
- Temporomandibular dysfunction: Pain and dysfunction in the jaw joint.

These indications are based on clinical studies and observations on the ability of dry needling to deactivate PGMs and reduce pain in various areas of the body.

1.3. Precautions in PS.

The hazards associated with dry needling (DP) are rare and their likelihood is low, especially if proper precautions are taken. However, it is essential that the physical therapist assess the risks versus the benefits of the technique, using his or her clinical judgment on a case-by-case basis. Non-invasive treatment should be considered to achieve the desired goals. The following are precautions to be taken into account (9, 10, 11).

1.3.1. Pain.

Pain is one of the most common adverse effects during trigger point treatment using PS. This pain can be severe when a local spasm response is elicited upon needle insertion. Although one study indicates a mean visual analog scale (VAS) pain of 5.25, clinical experience suggests that pain can often exceed 7 points. Post puncture pain can be significant, but is usually temporary and subsides within a few hours. A distinction should be made between post-puncture pain and referred pain that the patient was already experiencing. In research, it has been found that almost all patients undergoing PS report some post-puncture pain, although this is usually considered more tolerable compared to previous pain. Most of these symptoms are transient and do not usually cause serious complications (9, 10, 11).

1.3.2. Problems with needles

The use of needles in PS can lead to complications such as bending, jamming, breaking or getting lost. These problems are relatively common, but usually have minor consequences. Broken or forgotten needles are less common, although they can have serious consequences. To prevent needles from getting stuck or bent, it is crucial that the physical therapist maintains good control and has good technique. In rare cases, there may be incidents of forgotten needles in the patient, which could carry risks, so it is advisable to keep an accurate count of the needles used (9, 10, 11).

1.3.3. Pneumothorax.

Pneumothorax is a serious but rare complication that can arise from acupuncture or PS. It consists of the accumulation of air in the pleural cavity, which can lead to lung collapse. Although it is a potential risk, its occurrence is rare and can usually be prevented by proper anatomical knowledge and careful needling techniques. It is advisable to avoid performing deep punctures on both sides of the chest in the same session and to consider the use of ultrasound or alternative manual techniques if there are doubts about the safe performance of PS. Continuous training and attention to technique are essential to minimize these risks (9, 10, 11).

1.3.4. Vascular lesions in PS.

Dry needling is a technique that, although effective for the treatment of various muscular conditions, carries the risk of causing vascular injury. Understanding the anatomy of the vascular system is essential to avoid complications. At the start of the procedure, the physical therapist should be aware of the location of the major vessels and, as far as possible, palpate the pulses. However, some peripheral vessels are difficult to identify, which can complicate the technique. When a needle punctures a blood vessel, the patient usually feels a prick or stinging sensation, different from puncturing muscle tissue. Although these injuries may go unnoticed, they can result in serious bleeding. The most common complications include bleeding and hematoma formation. Although these are considered minor adverse effects, their implications can be significant. It is critical to distinguish between bleeding that occurs in muscle tissue and superficial bleeding that affects vessels at the cutaneous and subcutaneous level. The former can lead to alterations in local pH, affecting muscle function and causing additional discomfort. To manage any bleeding that arises, the therapist should apply firm pressure over the puncture site, maintaining it for at least 3 to 10 minutes, especially if a vessel is suspected to have been punctured (9, 10, 11, 12, 13).

Patients with vascular disease or those receiving anticoagulant therapy should be monitored with particular attention, as they are more prone to complications. In these cases, less invasive techniques should be adopted and extreme precautions should be taken, maintaining adequate hemostatic pressure after the procedure. Although severe complications, such as pseudoaneurysms or compartment syndromes, are rare, detailed anatomical knowledge and careful application of techniques can help prevent these situations (9, 10, 11, 12, 13).

1.3.5. Nerve lesions in PS for the peripheral nervous system (PNS).

In addition to vascular injuries, nerve injuries represent a significant risk in dry needling. To avoid these complications, it is vital that the physical therapist has a clear understanding of the anatomy and peripheral nerve pathways. Some areas of risk include muscles close to nerve structures, such as the piriformis and iliopsoas. One of the key precautions is not to insert the needle all the way to the handle, as the part closest to the skin is the most fragile and can cause complications if it gets close to a nerve. Needle insertion should be done slowly and carefully, watching for any signals the patient may provide. If the patient reports an electrical or stabbing sensation, this may indicate that a nerve has been pinched. In such a case, it is crucial to withdraw the needle and change the direction of insertion (9, 10, 11, 12, 13).

The use of ultrasound may be particularly beneficial in identifying nerve structures and minimizing the risk of accidental punctures. Although serious complications from nerve puncture are rare, cases of neuroparalysis and other adverse reactions have been documented. Studies have shown that among treated patients, mild reactions, such as tingling and paresthesia, have been reported. Fortunately, most of these cases are manageable, and patients tend to recover without significant complications. To mitigate the risk of nerve injury, it is crucial that the physical therapist exercise caution, adjusting his or her technique according to the sensations reported by the patient during the procedure (9, 10, 11, 12, 13).

1.3.6. Nerve injuries in PS for the central nervous system (CNS).

Nerve injuries represent one of the most critical complications in the practice of dry needling, especially when dealing with areas close to the central nervous system. Protection of the spinal cord is essential, especially when working with the deep paravertebral musculature or in the cervical spine muscles. To minimize the risk of contact with the spinal cord during dry needling, several recommendations should be followed (9, 10, 11, 12, 13):

- Needle length: It is important to use needles of adequate length. Needles of 40 mm are recommended for the cervical and thoracic regions, and 50 mm for the lumbar and sacral regions.
- Angle of insertion: When puncturing the deep paravertebral musculature, the needle should be inserted between 1 cm and 1.5 cm from the line of the spinous processes, with a craniocaudal inclination of approximately 10° to 15° along the spine. This prevents the needle from passing through the intervertebral spaces or facet joints, reducing the risk of epidural or subdural hematomas.

- Bone reference: Contact with the vertebral lamina, which acts as a barrier in front of the spinal canal, should be sought. This helps to confirm that the different strata of the transverse spinous muscles have been crossed. If the needle is introduced beyond the expected distances from the bone, the direction of the puncture should be adjusted.
- Precautions in the suboccipital triangle: In this area, bounded by the posterior greater rectus abdominis, superior oblique and inferior oblique muscles, it is vital to be especially careful. When working in this area or above the level of C2, the vertebral artery is exposed and unprotected.
- Patient sensations: During needle insertion, slow entry is crucial. The patient should be informed to report if he/she feels an electrical sensation, which may indicate nerve contact.

Although serious adverse reactions due to contact with the central nervous system are rare, there are documented cases. A study by Ernst et al. reported six adverse events, including (14, 15):

- Cervical spinal cord injury, resulting in a permanent deficit.
- Subarachnoid hemorrhage with no information on treatment or recovery.
- Epidural hematoma that recovered completely.
- Three cases related to broken needle fragments causing complications that were resolved surgically.
- Peuker et al. reviewed the literature and found ten cases of spinal cord or nerve root injuries, as well as cases of arachnoiditis and subarachnoid hemorrhages during acupuncture sessions. In their review, no vertebral artery injuries were found.

The chances of causing central nervous system injury are remote if safety recommendations are followed, which include slow needle entry and proper choice of needle length, as well as maintaining suggested angles of inclination and avoiding puncture above C2.

1.3.7. Visceral lesions in PS.

The most common visceral injury in dry needling is pneumothorax. Some muscles are in close proximity to abdominal viscera, which may cause unintentional injuries when treating muscles such as the psoas, quadratus lumborum or abdominal musculature. Although these events are rare, some have been documented (13, 14, 15):

- A needle fragment lodged in the kidney.
- A retroperitoneal hematoma.
- A renal complication following urinary bladder injury.
- A case of pancreatitis due to direct puncture.

In addition to the risks associated with pneumothorax, there is the potential for more serious injury, such as cardiac tamponade. The latter involves the accumulation of blood or fluid in the space between the myocardium and the pericardium, which can compromise cardiac function and be fatal if action is not taken quickly. In some cases, the needle has passed through the sternum due to a malformation known as sternal foramen, present in 5-8% of the population.

To avoid visceral complications, it is essential to have a good knowledge of the anatomy of the area and to adopt rigorous aseptic measures. Although there are few documented cases of significant visceral injury, it is essential to be aware of the risk of infection, which is the most common complication in this setting.

1.3.8. Infections.

The risk of infection in dry needling is considerable for both the patient and the physical therapist in the event of an accidental puncture with a used needle. Although the risk of infection is generally low, it is crucial to follow proper protocols to minimize this risk.

Considering the risk of infection to the patient when inserting a needle into the body, there is an inherent risk of infection. It is estimated that about 1,000 bacteria inhabit each square centimeter of skin, with more numerous bacteria in the underlying ducts and glands. However, these bacteria have little potential to cause infection, as illustrated in the work of Dann (68), who reported no infections after more than 5,000 injections without skin preparation. Wit et al (69). documented local infections in 0.014% of the 230,000 patients studied. In the review by Ernst et al. 38 serious infections were reported, especially septic arthritis and psoas abscesses, all of which were satisfactorily treated. Zhang et al (70). reported cases of bacterial and viral infections, emphasizing that these are generally due to bad practices, such as the use of reused and poorly sterilized needles.

To prevent infections in the physical therapist due to accidental punctures, should be considered (14, 15, 16):

- Careful needle handling: Avoid reinserting the needle into the guide tube in an unsafe manner and be careful when performing clamp punctures.
- Safe disposal: Take care when disposing of needles in specific containers to avoid accidental punctures.

By following these guidelines, the risk of complications associated with dry needling can be significantly reduced for both the patient and the physical therapist.

To minimize the risk of infection, the following precautions should be taken (17, 18, 19):

- Hand washing: Before performing the puncture, it is crucial to wash hands thoroughly with soap and water or a hydroalcoholic solution, even if gloves are used.
- Disinfection of the area: Although there is no consensus on its efficacy, it is recommended to clean the puncture site with 70° alcohol to reduce the number of germs.
- Use of sterile needles: Needles should be sterile and for single use only. They should never be reused for different treatments, even for the same patient.
- Careful handling of the needle: Handle the needle from the handle and avoid touching the part that will come into contact with the patient, unless absolutely necessary.
- Proper disposal of needles: Needles should be deposited in a specific container for biocontaminated material and replaced when the indicated limit is reached.
- Use of gloves: The use of latex or nitrile gloves is recommended, as they reduce the possibility of contagion in case of accidental puncture.

1.3.9. Vegetative reactions.

Vegetative reactions are common after puncture and may include vasovagal syncope, which is the most common adverse effect. They occur most frequently when the patient is in an upright position. Other symptoms include dizziness, sweating, tachycardia, and changes in blood pressure. Performing the puncture in the decubitus position is essential to prevent syncope and minimize the risk of injury in case of fainting (18, 19).

1.3.10. Puncture in pregnancy.

Caution should be exercised when performing punctures in pregnant women due to the possibility of miscarriage and misperceptions of causality by the patient or family members. It is recommended to avoid invasive techniques and opt for less aggressive methods, unless necessary. There is no scientific evidence to support the existence of "forbidden points" in acupuncture that could induce abortion. However, the risks should be considered (17, 18, 19).

1.3.11. Needle accidents in PS.

In the practice of PS, various needle accidents can occur, and it is crucial to know how to handle them properly. The most common accidents and their respective handling maneuvers are described below (14, 15, 16, 17):

- Bent needle: The needle may bend if the patient performs an intense muscular contraction while the needle is inserted. The needle should be withdrawn down to the subcutaneous tissue. Check if the needle is bent, if so, dispose of it properly to avoid risks of unwanted insertion or breakage.
- Stuck needle: The needle may get stuck in the skin or muscle. For its management we should ask the patient to relax as much as possible, try to extract the needle every 10-15 seconds, give soft blows on the skin around the needle and scrape the needle handle with the fingernail and try to extract it slowly. If the needle is very fixed, try to pinch the skin fold where it is inserted, to free it a little more and then try to pull it out. If the needle is stuck due to muscle spasm, two superficial needles can be inserted on both sides to help release the spasm.
- Blunt needle: Discard the needle immediately, as it may increase pain during manipulation.
- Broken needle: Inform the patient to remain calm to prevent the needle from penetrating deeper. Mark a circle around the insertion

site for reference. If a piece of needle is exposed, attempt to remove it with forceps. If no fragments are exposed, apply pressure to the surrounding skin to facilitate removal with forceps. If it cannot be removed in consultation, specialized medical attention will be required for surgical removal.

- Important considerations:
    - Needle quality: Always use needles with the European Community quality seal.
    - Insertion length: Always keep a margin of 0.5 cm to 1 cm of needle outside the skin to facilitate its removal in case of emergency.

These accidents can be serious, so it is essential that physical therapists practicing dry needling are well informed and prepared to handle them properly.

1.4. Contraindications in PS.

It is essential to know the absolute and relative contraindications, as well as the special precautions in the practice of PS. A complete evaluation of the patient should be performed to detect possible risks and diseases that may influence the treatment. PS should be avoided in the following situations (20, 21, 21, 22, 23):

- Absolute contraindications:
    - Needle phobia.
    - Patient refusal due to fear or beliefs.
    - Inability to give consent (cognitive, communication or age-related problems).
    - Medical emergencies or acute conditions.
    - Areas with lymphedema, due to increased risk of infection.
    - Other medical reasons that advise against PS.

- Relative contraindications

Once absolute contraindications have been ruled out, the clinician must assess the appropriateness of the treatment, considering the clinical history and the potential benefits versus risks. Some relative contraindications include:

- Tendency to hemorrhage: Patients with hemophilia, thrombocytopenia or on anticoagulant therapy require special attention.
- Immune system compromise: Those with immunosuppressive diseases (HIV, cancer, etc.) or under immunosuppressive treatment are at higher risk of infection.
- Vascular diseases: They may predispose to hematomas, hemorrhages and infections.
- Diabetes: Affects the regenerative capacity and circulation, increasing the risk of infections and hindering healing.
- Pregnancy: Caution should be exercised, especially in the first trimester, due to potential risks.

- Other special precautions:
  - Children: Parental or guardian consent is required, and deep PS should be avoided in children under 13-15 years of age.
  - Weakened or fragile patients: They may not tolerate the treatment adequately.
  - Epilepsy: Patients should not be left unsupervised while the needles are in place.
  - Psychological state: Anxiety or stress may interfere with tolerance to treatment.
  - Allergies: Especially to metals in needles (nickel, chromium) or latex in gloves.
  - Use of medications: Those that may affect the patient's immune system, coagulation or emotional stability should be taken into account.

In case of doubt about the patient's suitability, the treatment should be reconsidered or discarded to avoid risks.

1.5. Safety conditions.

Dry needling (SP) is an invasive procedure used in physical therapy and other disciplines to treat pain and muscle dysfunction. However, as a treatment involving the insertion of needles into tissues, it carries risks that are different from those associated with noninvasive therapies. Therefore, this section will focus on the safety of dry needling, addressing the considerations necessary to ensure the health of both patients and health professionals involved in its application. SP can be divided into two categories: superficial dry needling (SDP) and trigger point dry needling (TPDS). Each of these techniques has its own particularities and associated risks. It is essential that both healthcare professionals and patients understand the nature of these risks. According to the World Health Organization (WHO), the well-being of the patient is the highest priority, but it is also crucial to care for the health and safety of the practitioners and others who may be involved in the treatment (24, 25, 26).

The risks associated with PSPG are significant and may include hematoma, pneumothorax, infection, internal tissue injury and bleeding. The term "adverse effect" (AE) is used to describe any negative effect that may arise from a treatment, regardless of its severity. The classification of AEs can range from mild, which are brief and reversible, to severe, which may require hospitalization or result in significant disabilities or even death of the patient. Although the scientific literature still lacks comprehensive studies on PSPG-specific AEs, clinical experience suggests that serious adverse effects are infrequent. However, further research is essential to quantify these risks and provide a sound basis for informed patient consent (24, 25, 26).

Several studies have investigated the safety of acupuncture and have found that, although there are adverse effects, the incidence of serious events is low. For example, one study that analyzed 32,000 treatments performed by British physiotherapists and physicians found that most adverse effects were of low severity and often reversible. Other studies have shown a similar frequency of adverse effects in large cohorts of patients receiving acupuncture treatment, with bleeding and pain at the puncture site being the most common adverse effects (24, 25, 26).

However, it is important for healthcare professionals to be aware of the potential risks and adverse effects associated with any technique they use, including PSPG. Ongoing training and education on anatomy and needling techniques are crucial to minimize the risk of complications. Physical therapists must be proactive in identifying potential adverse effects and educating the patient about these risks. This includes the importance of informed consent, where patients should be informed not only about the benefits of treatment, but also about potential adverse effects (24, 25, 26).

1.5.1. Hand hygiene.

Dry needling (D&C) is an invasive procedure that carries certain risks, including the risk of healthcare-associated infections. The agents causing these infections are diverse and include bacteria such as Staphylococcus and E. coli, viruses such as hepatitis B and C, human immunodeficiency virus (HIV), fungi such as Candida albicans, protozoa such as toxoplasma and prions that can cause diseases such as Creutzfeldt-Jakob disease (27).

To better understand the transmission of infectious diseases, it is useful to refer to the concept of the chain of infection, which is made up of six essential elements: an infectious agent, a reservoir (the area where the agent is found), an exit gate (the means by which the agent leaves the infected), a means of transmission, an entry gate (the way in which the agent enters the new host) and, finally, a susceptible host that can be infected. This model is fundamental for developing effective prevention strategies (27, 28).

Standard precautions, developed and published by the Centers for Disease Control and Prevention, are a set of clinical guidelines designed to prevent the transmission of infectious agents. Their main objective is to interrupt the chain of infection by focusing on the mode of transmission, the gateway of entry and the susceptible host. These precautions require healthcare professionals to assume that any person can potentially be infected or colonized by microorganisms that can be transmitted in the healthcare setting. Therefore, they must apply a series of work practices to minimize the risk of contamination. These practices include critical aspects such as hand hygiene, glove use, proper skin preparation, safe handling of needles and medical waste, as well as the prevention of needlestick injuries (28).

Hand hygiene is considered the most important intervention to prevent the transmission of infections. Recommendations related to this practice have been classified into three categories, according to the level of evidence supporting them (29):

- Category I refers to solid evidence supported by experimental, clinical or epidemiological studies.
- Category II includes results suggestive of clinical or epidemiological studies.
- Category III is based on the recommendations of healthcare experts based on their experience.

To carry out effective hand hygiene, it is essential that the nails are short and perfectly manicured. False nails, nail extensors and the use of varnish or nail polish should be avoided. In addition, it is advisable to remove any type of jewelry or costume jewelry from the hands and wrists, except for the wedding ring, and the sleeves of shirts should be short or rolled up. Hand decontamination is preferably performed with a suitable soap and water, although if the hands are visibly clean of contaminants, an appropriate gel or alcohol solution may be used. Hand decontamination is recommended in several specific situations, such as when hands are visibly soiled, before and after each patient contact, at the beginning and end of each work shift, after removing gloves, when leaving a contaminated area, after using soiled equipment or materials, after performing personal body functions, and before handling food (28, 29).

Attention to hand decontamination technique is crucial because, despite its apparent simplicity, it is common for healthcare professionals to apply incorrect techniques. Conventional hand washing with soap can remove visible soil, but is often less effective in preventing microorganism activity. On the other hand, alcoholic solutions for hand washing have been shown to be more effective in this regard. Antimicrobial soaps prove to be more effective than conventional soaps, achieving a statistically significant reduction in microbial activity. However, the use of alcohol in gels is superior to antimicrobial or mild non-alcoholic soaps (30, 31).

Recommendations for proper hand washing with soap are as follows: first, wet hands with water; then apply an adequate amount of soap as directed by the manufacturer; rub hands vigorously for at least 15 seconds, making sure to cover all hand and finger surfaces; rinse hands with water; dry with a good quality disposable paper towel; use the towel to turn off the faucet and dispose of it in a bucket with a pedal; and avoid using hot water, as it can increase skin dryness and contribute to dermatitis (30, 31).

Alternatively, hands can be decontaminated with an alcohol solution or hand gel, as long as they are visibly clean. However, it is important to note that organic material can inactivate these solutions, so if the hands are soiled, they should be washed beforehand. It is recommended that the alcohol solution have a concentration of approximately 70% isopropanol, ethanol or n-propanol, as higher concentrations may increase the risk of dryness and dermatitis. It is suggested that hands be washed with soap every 5-10 applications of alcoholic gel to reconstitute the skin emollients (30, 31).

Given that healthcare professionals may perform up to 30 hand washes in a single work shift, there is a significant risk of skin irritation and dermatitis. Irritant dermatitis is a non-immunologic inflammatory response of the skin to an external agent, which can make the skin more susceptible to colonization by microorganisms. Therefore, prevention and treatment of all forms of dermatitis are crucial to the safety of both patients and healthcare professionals. To prevent occupational dermatitis in the healthcare setting, it is recommended to follow the manufacturer's instructions on the use of hand hygiene products, choose products with a low irritant potential and use emollients whenever possible. It is also important to pay attention to feedback from professionals on the products they use, as well as to use appropriate hand lotions that help maintain hydration and restore skin lipids (27, 28, 29).

1.5.2. Gloves.

The use of gloves is essential in dry needling because they prevent contact with blood and other body fluids, especially in the face of the frequent risk of hemorrhage. Although some argue that gloves may affect touch sensitivity, their use is mandatory according to regulations, and they must be disposable after each use. In the case of latex allergies, nitrile gloves are preferred. In addition, after their removal, it is necessary to wash the hands to avoid bacterial proliferation. Disinfection of the patient's skin before puncture is generally not necessary if it is visibly clean, following WHO recommendations. However, in some countries the use of disinfectants, such as isopropyl alcohol, is required, especially in areas with a higher risk of moisture accumulation. For immunocompromised patients, more rigorous preparation with specific disinfectant solutions, such as 2% iodine in alcohol, is recommended. Needles and other medical waste should be disposed of according to local regulations, using special sharps containers. These should be easily accessible during the procedure, but out of reach of children, and should not be filled above the safety line to avoid accidents (30, 31, 32, 33).

Puncture wounds (LP) are a common risk for healthcare professionals. These injuries can transmit dangerous pathogens such as HIV and hepatitis B and C viruses. Although the risk is lower with solid filament needles, it is crucial to maintain proper hygiene and waste disposal practices. In the event of an LP, the wound should be washed immediately, the incident reported, and medical attention sought. To prevent these injuries, practitioners should monitor needle use and disposal carefully, avoid interruptions, and work under optimal conditions. In addition, they should be vaccinated against hepatitis A and B. Not only practitioners, but also patients and their families are at risk if needles are not properly disposed of, so it is essential to maintain a safe environment (30, 31, 32, 33).

1.5.3. Safety during the procedure.

Dry needling (DP) is an invasive procedure that may be associated with adverse effects. Patient education and good communication with the clinician are essential for safe and effective practice. Pain after dry needling, known as post-treatment discomfort (MTT), is common and can last from 1 to 4 days. This discomfort is more common with deep trigger point dry needling (DTP) and less likely with superficial dry needling (SD). Patients should be informed about these possible discomforts to avoid unnecessary concerns. It is important to communicate with the patient to adjust the treatment according to their tolerance. If the patient experiences persistent, sharp pain during needle insertion, the needle should be removed and repositioned to a nearby area. Sharp or electrical pain may indicate that the needle has touched a nerve or blood vessel, in which case it should be withdrawn immediately and pressure applied to control possible bleeding (26, 34).

Hematoma is a frequent adverse effect. To reduce its occurrence, it is essential to avoid puncturing blood vessels and to apply manual pressure after needle removal. In case of skin bleeding, pressure should be used and ice should be applied if necessary. Fainting may occur during treatment due to factors such as pain, stress or needle phobia. To prevent this, the patient should be treated in a lying position. Maintain constant communication and avoid aggressive techniques. If the patient shows signs of dizziness or sweating, remove the needle and consider elevating the legs (26, 34).

Although the risk of infection is low, it is important to follow strict hygiene protocols. The puncture site should be inspected before and after treatment to identify possible signs of infection (pain, redness, fever, etc.). In punctures close to the thorax, there is a low but potential risk of pneumothorax. If suspected, the patient should be taken to the emergency department. Some patients may experience fatigue or drowsiness after SP. They should be warned not to drive or operate machinery until these symptoms disappear (26, 34).

2. DRY NEEDLING TECHNIQUES.

2.1. Classification and modalities of the PS.

Dry needling (DP) is a technique used to treat myofascial trigger points (MTrPs) and has different modalities. These can be classified according to several criteria, such as the tool used, the type of stimulation, the depth of needle insertion, the conceptual model on which the technique is based or the practitioner performing the technique. However, the most commonly used criterion is the depth of the needle in relation to the PGM. There are two broad categories: superficial dry needling (SDP) and deep dry needling (DDP). In PSS, the needle does not penetrate the PGM, while in PSP the needle penetrates the PGM. Regarding the modalities, the best known are:

For PSS is the Peter Baldry technique, in which the needle is inserted into the subcutaneous tissues without reaching the PGM. This technique proved effective in reducing pain and hyperalgesia associated with PGMs, even in deep muscles. It is characterized by leaving the needle in the skin for 30 seconds, and if pain persists, the insertion time can be extended or additional stimulation can be applied (4, 35, 36).

Another technique is Fu subcutaneous puncture, which requires specific needles and seeks to mobilize the needle in the subcutaneous tissue at a certain distance from the PGM. This movement is repeated several times, and the catheter used can be left inside the body for several hours (35, 36, 37, 38, 39).

Regarding PSP, Hong's rapid entry and exit technique, which seeks to provoke local spasm responses (REL) by rapidly inserting and withdrawing the needle from the MMP, stands out. RELs are an indicator of treatment efficacy, and the number of insertions depends on patient tolerance (35, 36, 37, 38, 39).

Another technique that can be found is Gunn's intramuscular stimulation. This diagnostic and therapeutic approach focuses on the treatment of chronic pain, suggesting that myofascial trigger points (MTrPs) are the result of radiculopathies or alterations of the nervous system. It uses acupuncture needles inserted and manipulated with an injector, making rapid entries and exits and twists in both directions to elicit an endorphin release response (REL) or referred pain. If the pain does not disappear or increases, it is recommended to discontinue the technique (35, 36, 37, 38, 39).

The rapid entry and exit technique with rotation is the adaptation of the multiple insertion technique, designed to facilitate needle insertion without bending. The needle is rotated on insertion and withdrawal, and is further detailed in the corresponding chapter (35, 36, 37, 38, 39).

The needle twisting technique is proposed as a less aggressive alternative for sensitive patients. It is based on the manipulation of the needle by twisting, a classic practice in traditional Chinese medicine. Efficacy is evaluated through REL or referred pain, which indicates the correct localization of the PGM. If relief is not achieved, the direction of the needle can be changed and the procedure repeated (35, 36, 37, 38, 39).

For the mini-scalpel needle deep dry needling technique is compared to conventional acupuncture needles and self-stretching exercises, this technique has shown significantly superior results in the treatment of PGM. The thicker miniscalpel needle with a sharp tip is used in cases that do not respond to other treatments. However, more evidence is needed to justify its widespread use due to its more aggressive nature (35, 36, 37, 38, 39).

With respect to dry electropuncture, it acts through several mechanisms that justify its efficacy. Firstly, it is postulated that the electric current has the capacity to cause myocyte destruction around the needle, in addition to the mechanical injury already caused by the needle itself. However, it is important to note that this theory still needs to be validated by further research to determine the extent of this destruction and the dose required for it to occur. Another interesting mechanism is the washout of sensitizing substances. During the application of dry electropuncture, small but visible muscle contractions are achieved by slightly exceeding the excitomotor threshold. These contractions can facilitate a "washing out" effect on the sensitizing substances accumulated in the area, similar to what is observed in the relaxation techniques (REL) used in dry needling. In addition, the contractions provoked by the electric current also contribute to the local stretching of shortened sarcomeres at myofascial trigger points (MTrPs). This stretching helps to normalize muscle length, which in turn improves muscle function. Taken together, these mechanisms make dry electropuncture a promising tool in the treatment of muscle dysfunctions (35, 36, 37, 37, 38, 39).

2.2. Mechanisms and effects of PS.

2.2.1. Mechanisms of action of PS.

Superficial dry needling (SDP) and deep dry needling (DDP) are two techniques used in the treatment of myofascial pain, and although both involve the insertion of a needle, their mechanisms of action are different. PSS focuses on tissue surface stimulation without reaching myofascial trigger points (MTrPs), which leads to its effects not being justified solely by mechanical factors. Instead, it seeks to understand its efficacy through neurophysiology and endogenous mechanisms that modulate pain (4).

One of the most relevant mechanisms in PSS is the stimulation of A-beta nerve fibers, which are activated when the needle is inserted into the tissues above the PGM. This can block the transmission of nociceptive impulses coming from type IV muscle fibers, responsible for myofascial pain. This action can be direct, via inhibitory interneurons in the spinal cord, or indirect, via descending systems that use opioids, serotonin and noradrenaline to inhibit pain perception. In addition, diffuse inhibitory control of nociception is activated, which can also be activated by peripheral C-fibers, contributing to pain reduction (4).

The gate control theory, proposed by Melzack and Wall, suggests that stimulation of large-diameter A-beta nerve fibers closes the "gate" to pain transmission to the central nervous system. Although it has been revised over time, the essence of this theory persists and is considered fundamental to understanding how PSS can reduce pain perception. On the other hand, action on the autonomic nervous system is another mechanism under investigation. It has been found that this system can modulate the activity of PGMs, and animal studies suggest that sympathetic stimulation can increase the release of acetylcholine, which could contribute to decreased tension and improve the mobility of affected muscles (39).

With respect to PSP, this technique not only induces PSS, but also targets PGMs, eliciting responses that translate into additional mechanisms of action. One of the proposed mechanisms is the "washout" of sensitizing substances in the PGMs. By eliciting an endorphin release response (REL) via puncture, it has been shown to decrease the concentrations of compounds such as bradykinin and substance P, which are responsible for sensitization and perpetuation of pain. This "washout" may be related to an increase in blood flow that facilitates the elimination of these substances and improves motor plate physiology. Another mechanism of PSP is the elevation of pH in the PGM area, which is crucial, as an acidic pH is associated with pain sensitization. Studies show that after REL provocation, the pH of active PGMs rises, approaching normal muscle levels, which could help normalize motor plate function (3, 39, 40).

In addition, it has been proposed that stimulation of the PGM may interrupt the "PGM circuit", restoring the control that the central nervous system exerts over the affected area and contributing to the release of endorphins. It has also been observed that the puncture may cause mechanical laceration of myocytes and motor plates, which may lead to regeneration and functional reorganization of the affected tissues (3, 39, 40).

Local stretching of contracted cytoskeletal structures is another mechanism that has been suggested, where the needle causes a stretch that may contribute to the normalization of sarcomere length, improving muscle function. Finally, the effects on blood flow and anti-inflammatory action following puncture are additional mechanisms that highlight the complexity of PSP. It has been observed that this technique can improve oxygenation and blood flow in muscles, which is essential to counteract the hypoxia that characterizes PGMs (3, 39, 40).

In summary, PSS and PSP present a number of mechanisms of action that go beyond the merely mechanical, involving complex interactions between the nervous, vascular and immune systems, which explains their analgesic and therapeutic effects in the treatment of myofascial pain. These findings invite further research on the efficacy and underlying mechanisms of these techniques, especially in terms of their comparison with placebo and their possible combination with other treatment modalities.

2.2.2. Effects on connective tissue.

In dry needling, thin, filiform needles are used to interact with the connective tissue of the body. The efficacy of these techniques is related to the small diameter of the needles (generally less than 300 mm), which allows for a specific interaction with the tissue, creating what is known as a "ball or swirl" of collagen around the needle. This phenomenon occurs when the needles are rotated, causing the collagen bundles to adhere and rotate with them, which increases the mechanical bond between the needle and the tissue. The mechanism of action is realized by (3, 39, 40, 41, 42):

- Needle rotation: By rotating the needle, a specific stretching of the connective tissue is generated, mainly affecting the subcutaneous and intermuscular layers, with minimal impact on the skin.
- Sustained stretch: When the needle is left in place after rotation, the collagen ball does not immediately unravel, allowing localized stretching to be maintained for several minutes.
- Measurement and quantification: Techniques, such as robotic acupuncture puncture and ultrasound elastography, have been developed to quantify connective tissue tangles and tissue displacements induced by needle manipulation.

Connective tissue constantly responds to mechanical forces, and this type of stimulation can induce viscoelastic responses depending on its composition and organization. Sustained stretching of the tissue beyond its usual range can lead to (43, 39, 40, 41, 42):

- Viscoelastic relaxation: Initially the tension in the tissue is reduced, followed by a molecular reorganization in the collagen matrix that restores the tension balance.
- Alterations in fibroblasts: These changes in cell shape (flattening and expansion) are active responses that may result in remodeling of the cytoskeleton and further reduction of tissue tension.

Although there is abundant evidence to suggest that manual needle stimulation influences the nervous system, there is still little knowledge about the mechanical link between the needle and the nervous system. The possibility that collagen coiling is an important mechanism for the transmission of mechanical signals is supported by studies where needle manipulation loses analgesic efficacy when the collagen-tissue link is disrupted. Some studies suggest a correspondence between acupuncture meridians and connective tissue, indicating that acupuncture points may be located in areas of denser or deeper connective tissue, which could explain differences in resistance to needle withdrawal at these points compared to control points (39, 40, 41, 42, 43).

2.2.3. Effects on muscle fascia.

The term "myofascial" was coined by Janet Travell in relation to trigger points (TP), which are hypersensitive areas in muscles that can generate referred pain. However, the scientific literature and Travell and Simons' seminal texts on PGs have tended to present muscles as isolated, self-contained structures with clearly defined origins and functions. This simplistic view does not reflect the complexity of the interrelationship between muscles and the fascial structures that surround them, a relationship that is crucial to understanding the etiology of myofascial pain. Fascia is classified into two main types: superficial fascia and deep fascia. Superficial fascia is composed of lax connective tissue, which lies just beneath the skin and contains collagen, elastin and adipose tissue. In contrast, the deep fascia is denser and surrounds muscles, nerves, blood vessels and organs, lacking adipose tissue. The separation between the deep fascia and the muscles is accomplished through a layer of lax connective tissue containing hyaluronan, a compound that facilitates sliding between the layers, essential to allow proper movement and reduce friction during muscle contraction (39, 40, 41, 42, 43).

The fascial layers surrounding the muscle are composed of epimysium, perimysium and endomysium. The epimysium envelops specific muscles and connects directly to the perimysium, which bundles bundles of muscle fibers. In turn, the endomysium wraps each muscle fiber individually, playing a vital role in flexibility and force transmission along the myofibrils. Tension in the deep fascia is maintained by numerous muscle insertions, allowing the muscles to distribute some of their contractile forces to the fascial structures. This interaction not only increases joint stability, but also facilitates coordinated movement between different muscle groups (39, 40, 41, 42, 43).

An interesting finding is that, although some muscles may have strong mechanical connections with their agonist muscles, force transmission is not always influenced by changes in the length of these muscles. This suggests that the mechanisms used to transmit force may vary between different muscles, further complicating our understanding of muscle and fascial function. In the context of dry needling, which involves inserting a needle into a PG, it is critical to consider how this procedure affects not only the PGs, but also the surrounding fascial structures. Dry needling resembles an injection treatment, and since the needle must pass through superficial and deep fascia to reach the PG, it is essential to investigate how these treatments interact with fascial structures. Langevin and colleagues have proposed that the rotation of solid filament needles may cause internal stretching in the tissues. They also suggested that there may be coupling between the needle and body tissues, possibly mediated by surface tensions and electrical attraction, although the latter may be relatively weak (42).

Myofascial pain is associated with the presence of tight bands, which are palpable perpendicular to the direction of the muscle fibers. This raises the hypothesis that restrictions in the fascia, particularly in the perimysium, could contribute to the formation of these tight bands. Indeed, the perimysium has been observed to respond to changes in mechanical tension more than other intramuscular connective tissues, indicating a significant relationship between fascia and the experience of pain. Recent research has suggested that modifications in lax connective tissue density in deep fascia, as well as hyaluronan hydrodynamics, may be contributing factors to the development of myofascial pain (39, 40, 41, 42, 43).

Despite the importance of the topic, research on the role of fascia in PGs and myofascial pain has been sparse. Many questions remain unanswered, such as what are the effects of dry needling on fascial adhesions, areas of densification, scar tissue, and the development of strength and flexibility. There is an urgent need for studies that define in detail the interactions between PGs, muscles and fasciae to better understand their role in myofascial pain. Understanding the relationship between fascia and trigger points is critical to developing more effective treatments. The interconnection between muscles and fascia is complex and must be integrated into clinical practice to adequately address pain associated with PGs. By recognizing the crucial role of fascial structures, healthcare professionals can optimize their therapeutic approach, potentially improving outcomes for their patients (39, 40, 41, 42, 43).

2.3. Principles and application procedures for correct practice in PS.

2.3.1. Medical history.

The medical history is the first essential step in ensuring effective treatment. In this process, the physical therapist must perform a thorough collection of patient information. This includes the medical history, documenting pre-existing conditions, past surgical interventions and any previous physiotherapeutic treatment received. In addition, it is essential to record current symptoms, detailing their nature, duration and location. A thorough physical assessment should also be carried out, analyzing range of motion, muscle strength and identification of trigger points. This information will allow the physiotherapist to decide the best therapeutic intervention to follow (44, 45).

2.3.2. Patient information and consent.

Once the clinical history has been collected, it is crucial to inform the patient about the proposed treatment. This information process should include a clear explanation of the dry needling technique: how it is performed and what the intended goals are. In addition, the physiotherapist should list the advantages of the treatment, such as pain reduction and improved mobility. However, it is also important to discuss the drawbacks and associated risks, such as post-procedural pain or possible bruising. By ensuring that the patient is well informed, a relationship of trust is created that will facilitate the process. Given the invasive nature of dry needling, it is essential to obtain the patient's consent. This consent must be informed, which means that the patient must fully understand what the procedure entails. It is recommended that, after explanation of the technique and its possible effects, the patient sign a consent form. This document not only ensures that the patient has understood the procedure, but also protects both the patient and the physical therapist in case of any eventuality (46, 47).

We must make a statement that I have received clear and understandable verbal information about the procedure to be performed on me and, furthermore, that I have read this document. All my doubts have been answered and I understand all the information provided. Therefore, I voluntarily give my consent for the physiotherapist specialized in dry needling to perform this technique on me. I also understand that I may withdraw my consent at any time without explanation. I will be offered a copy of this document upon request (48, 49).

2.3.3. Hygiene.

Hygiene is a critical aspect in physical therapy practice, especially in invasive procedures. Prior to initiating the puncture, the physical therapist must comply with all established hygienic standards. This includes careful hand washing and, in many cases, the use of disposable gloves to create a barrier against any possible contamination. The patient's skin should also be disinfected in the area to be treated, using an appropriate antiseptic. The correct application of these rules ensures patient safety and reduces the risk of infection (50, 51).

2.3.4. Patient positioning.

Correct positioning of the patient is another vital aspect of a safe procedure. The physical therapist should ensure that the patient is in a comfortable prone position that allows easy access to the area to be treated. This position not only benefits the patient's comfort, but also allows the physical therapist to work more easily and safely. In addition, the use of cushions or supports can help ensure that the patient is as comfortable as possible during treatment (52, 53).

2.3.5. Diagnosis, localization and safe fixation of the PGM.

Before proceeding with the puncture, it is imperative to confirm the diagnosis and location of the muscle trigger point (MTrP). Without this step, the puncture could become an arbitrary procedure with unpredictable results. The physical therapist must ensure that the MTrP is correctly identified and fixed in a position that allows access during the puncture. This step is crucial, as it ensures that the treatment is specific and effective (54, 55).

2.3.6. Execution.

When the time comes to perform the puncture, it should be done with the greatest possible skill. Needle insertion should be done in a controlled manner, avoiding unnecessary depths to minimize risks. Throughout the process, it is essential to maintain constant communication with the patient, asking about their comfort and any symptoms they may be experiencing. This not only ensures that the patient feels safe, but also allows the physical therapist to adjust his or her technique as needed (54, 55).

2.3.7. Post-surgery care.

Finally, once the puncture has been performed, certain care must be taken to ensure the patient's well-being. It is essential to apply hemostasis techniques to stop any bleeding at the puncture site. In addition, clear instructions should be provided to the patient on how to care for the treated area and what activities to avoid after the procedure. Adequate follow-up is equally important; scheduling a subsequent appointment allows the effectiveness of the treatment to be evaluated and any side effects that may have arisen to be addressed (54, 55, 56, 57).

2.4. Injuries caused by PS.

Dry needling (DP) is a technique used to treat myofascial pain syndrome, and is based on the abnormally high release of acetylcholine, which generates localized muscle contractures. These contractures, located just below or within a few microns of the synaptic area, are known as "active sites" in functional studies and "contraction nodes" in histological analysis. The accumulation of these active sites forms a myofascial trigger point (MTrP), which can be detected by palpation. PS seeks to eliminate these MTrPs to relieve pain symptoms, but its application can also cause damage to muscle and nerve fibers. The needles used in PS have a diameter ranging from 0.16 mm to 0.45 mm, considerably larger than that of myocytes, which on average is 40 µm. Needle insertion causes focal injury to the myocytes, classified as a laceration. To date, there have been no studies on the cellular evolution of lesions caused by PS in muscles with PGM, so the available data come from experiments in healthy rodent muscles, specifically the levator atri longus muscle, subjected to multiple punctures (57, 58, 59).

Muscle injury caused by PS is characterized by localized mechanical damage, which begins with a phase of degeneration caused by the inflammatory response. This cleansing phase is responsible for eliminating cellular debris, which is subsequently replaced by muscle regeneration. These degeneration, regeneration and repair processes occur simultaneously, although they are described separately in the text. The rupture of the muscle fiber membrane allows water to enter the cell, which causes cellular products to be released into the extracellular medium. PS also affects the blood vessels, resulting in extravasation of blood into the injured area. Intracellular substances activate mast cells in muscle tissue, which release chemokines into the bloodstream, attracting inflammatory cells. Initially, neutrophils are the predominant cells, followed by monocytes that become macrophages, responsible for phagocytosis of cellular debris. This process is specific, since it affects only necrotic debris and preserves the basal lamina, which serves as a support for viable satellite cells in the formation of new myofibers (57, 58, 59).

The accumulation of water in the injured area causes inflammation of the cisterns of the sarcoplasmic system, which store calcium for muscle contraction. Overhydration of these cisternae causes their rupture, releasing calcium which activates localized contractions in the area of injury and also acts on calcium-dependent proteases (CANP), which degrade the contractile apparatus. Over time, muscle regeneration becomes more evident, limited to the injured area by the formation of a contraction band that acts as a "firewall". This band prevents the spread of damage along the myocyte, ensuring that the majority of the muscle fiber remains intact (57, 58, 59).

The process of muscle regeneration is based on the activation of satellite cells, which are muscle stem cells located under the basal lamina of myocytes. These cells are activated after injury, becoming myoblasts, which multiply and enrich their membrane with calcium channels. Subsequently, the myoblasts fuse to form myotubes, assembling the new contractile apparatus with the surviving ends of the injured myocyte. This process may take about 7 days in minor injuries such as those caused by PS, during which time the regenerated muscle fibers tend to be atrophic, being referred to as young or immature muscle fibers. As normal contractile activity resumes, these fibers acquire adequate trophism. As muscle regeneration proceeds, fibroblasts synthesize proteins and proteoglycans to restore the extracellular matrix, essential for connective tissue integrity. Fibroblasts, which are resident cells in the endomysium, are activated by both mechanical aggression and intracellular substances released. Initially, they produce type III collagen, followed by type I collagen, which is difficult to eliminate and is broken down only into small fragments. Muscle contraction facilitates this elimination, and from the seventh day post-puncture, the collagen is segmented, being phagocytosed by inflammatory cells. With time, the excess collagen is eliminated, restoring the pre-injury conditions (57, 58, 59).

PS can cause axonal injury, resulting in distal segment degeneration and loss of function due to activation of axonal calpains, which degrade neurofilaments. The inflammatory reaction, mediated by macrophages, facilitates phagocytosis of axonal debris. After phagocytosis of the distal segment, the reinnervation process begins, where intracellular factors and mitogens promote axonal growth to reconnect with the postsynaptic component. The rate of reinnervation is 1-3 mm/day, crucial to restore neuromuscular function. However, complications such as aberrant connections can occur, and success depends on the health of the microenvironment and management of inflammation (57, 58, 59).

Dry needling causes a clean lesion in the axon, which favors rapid reinnervation due to the proximity between the lesion site and the myocyte. The speed of reinnervation is linked to axoplasmic transport and preservation of the glial pathway, which facilitates the advancement of the axonal growth cone. Patient age is also an important factor, as regeneration tends to be impaired in older individuals. Although PS usually avoids damage to the active site of the nerve, it can affect muscle fibers outside the synaptic area. Studies in the levator auris longus muscle of mice have shown that, after multiple punctures, the inflammatory response intensifies in the first 24 hours, with almost complete muscle regeneration within 7 days. Intramuscular nerve injuries lead to rapid denervation of the postsynaptic component, followed by reinnervation within 3 days. In general, repetitive punctures do not adversely affect the processes of muscle regeneration and reinnervation (57, 58, 59).

3. PS OF NON-MYOFASCIAL TRIGGER POINTS (NMTP).

Dry needling (DP) refers to the insertion of a needle through the skin without the introduction of drugs, in contrast to infiltration which does involve the use of drugs. This chapter focuses on the PS of non-myofascial trigger points (NMTPs), while myofascial trigger points (MTrPs) are discussed in other chapters of the book. A classification of the different PS techniques is presented, followed by a definition of MTrPs and the most common treatment techniques (60, 61).

Theoretically, any spot that is painful to the touch and is not a PGM is classified as a PGNM. This includes (60, 61):

- Insertional trigger points in tendon attachment areas.
- Sore spots in sheaths, bursae, fasciae, and ligaments.
- Areas of injury due to trauma.
- Stitches in subcutaneous tissues.

PGNMs can be triggered by local spasm responses due to stimulation of an active PGM. Hong defines PGNMs as a set of sensitization foci, with sensitized nociceptors due to central or peripheral sensitization. PS at these foci can produce analgesia by hyperstimulation and relieve pain, sometimes using acupuncture points that are not painful (62, 63).

Regarding treatment, traditional Chinese acupuncture is one of the first techniques applied to treat PGNM, since many acupuncture points are Ah-Shi points, which are located in non-muscular tissues. When applying acupuncture, the needle can be rotated or electrical stimulation can be applied to increase efficacy. Other techniques in the treatment of PGNM include (62, 63):

- PS with multiple rapid insertions: Originally used by Travell to infiltrate PGMs, this technique involves multiple rapid needle insertions to localize and desensitize nociceptors. It seeks to stimulate a greater number of sensitized nociceptors by rapid movement, avoiding tissue damage and causing immediate pain relief.
- PS for soft tissue release: This technique focuses on soft tissue manipulation to release tension and pain.
- PS with electrostimulation: Combines PS with electrical stimulation to enhance the analgesic effect.

- Superficial PS: Applies PS to the surface of the skin, similar to acupuncture, although it generally does not provide complete immediate pain relief.
- PGNM PS, especially through the multiple rapid insertion technique, focuses on relieving pain by treating the underlying source of pain, rather than focusing solely on the PGM.

3.1. Mechanisms of PS in PGNM.

Dry needling (DP) is a therapeutic technique that uses needles to treat trigger points, with the aim of relieving pain. Several mechanisms have been proposed to explain how SP can achieve this relief (62, 63):

- Downstream pain inhibitory system: This system is an intrinsic mechanism of the body that controls pain. It is suggested that both hyperstimulation analgesia and disruption of the "PGM circuit" act through this system. According to Melzack, hyperstimulation analgesia is the main therapeutic mechanism of acupuncture for pain relief. During PS, local spasm responses (REL) are generated, which are essential for immediate and complete pain relief (39).
- Interruption of the vicious circle: Hong proposes that the main mechanism of PS is to interrupt the vicious circle of the PGM circuit, which could also include the connection of PGNMs to trigger point circuits in the spinal cord.
- Stimulation of nociceptors: When PS is performed, nerve impulses are sent to cells in the dorsal horn of the spinal cord, which can break the vicious circle of the PGM circuit. Vigorous stimulation of sensitive loci (sensitized nociceptors) is key to achieving optimal pain relief.

3.2. Application of the PS technique for PGNM.

The following practical considerations should be taken into account (64, 65):

- Type of needles: The use of hypodermic needles with the following sizes is recommended:
  - 0.50 mm x 40 mm for normal use.
  - 0.60 mm x 70 mm for thick or deep tissues.
  - 0.40 mm x 30 mm for thin and superficial tissues.

- Acupuncture needles can also be used, although they are more difficult to handle and require practice. The needles should be thicker than 0.30 mm.

- Insertion Technique: Before performing the puncture, it is essential to ensure that other non-invasive therapies have been explored and that any pathological lesions responsible for the pain have been removed. During the puncture the needle is directed towards the most sensitive region, moving rapidly inwards and outwards. Any lateral movement should be avoided, ensuring that the needle tip contacts as many sensitized nociceptors as possible. The needle insertion speed should be approximately 20-30 mm/s.
- Post-procedure: After puncture, compression should be applied to the penetration site to avoid excessive bleeding and reduce post-puncture pain.

3.3. Types of PS techniques in PGNM.

Regarding the types of techniques we can find (64, 65):

- Rapid entry and exit technique with rotation: Chou et al. have developed a recent technique known as "rapid entry and exit with rotation" using acupuncture needles. Because acupuncture needles are flexible and their small gauge makes rapid movement difficult, Chou incorporated needle rotation (coiling) to facilitate the movement in and out, preventing bending during the procedure. This technique is especially useful in people with fibromyalgia, as the small diameter of the needle minimizes tissue irritation, reducing pain and post-puncture discomfort, which often lasts several days in these patients. For its procedure the technique is performed with acupuncture needles. Rapid entries and exits are performed with simultaneous rotation of the needle to avoid bending.
- PS for soft tissue release: To treat chronic musculoskeletal problems that do not respond to physical therapy or infiltrations, surgical intervention or minimally invasive techniques are often required. Among these techniques is dry needling for soft tissue release. Lin's technique has developed a less invasive technique to release adherent soft tissues by using a blunt cannula to simultaneously inject hyaluronic acid and local anesthetic. Alternatively, a normal dry needle puncture can be used if applied slowly. With respect to the procedure the needle penetrates the skin and advances slowly into

the painful region. In addition, a lateral movement is performed to release soft tissue adhesions. The presence of pain or resistance to the movement of the needle indicates the location of the adhesions. Once the resistance decreases, the needle is withdrawn into the subcutaneous layer and redirected to penetrate in different trajectories to release the adherent tissues extensively. This technique is effective for releasing tendon adhesions, often related to insertional myofascial trigger points (MTrPs). The most common adhesions that can be treated include rotator cuff tendons, biceps brachii tendons, forearm extensor and flexor muscles at the elbow, and the quadriceps tendon and patellar ligament.

Dry needling techniques with rapid entry and exit with rotation, and dry needling for soft tissue release, are effective approaches to treat non-myofascial trigger points (NMTPs). These techniques can trigger hyperstimulation analgesia and, when performed properly, can relieve pain and release adhesions in tissues such as tendons, ligaments and fascia.

4. ***CLASSIFICATION AND PS IN THE PGM OF THE DIFFERENT MUSCULATURE.***

4.1. Musculature of the head.

4.1.1. Masseter.

- Symptoms and referred pain: The masseter muscle is multipenniform, meaning that its motor plates are distributed throughout the muscle, both in its central part and in the cranial and caudal insertions. PGMs can be found in different areas, which influences the referred pain patterns (67, 68):
  - Surface division:
    - Upper zone: Pain is projected to the maxilla, eyebrow, mandible, posterior oral mucosa and upper and lower molars.
    - Middle zone: Projects pain to the buccal and oral region, including the labial commissure and the upper and lower premolars and canines.
    - Lower area: Pain may radiate to the submandibular area and the posterior and inferior angle of the mandible.
  - Deep division: PGMs in this area may cause referred otalgia (ear pain not associated with otologic pathology) and affect the TMJ (temporomandibular joint), and may even cause tinnitus of myofascial origin. It can also radiate pain towards the anterior fascicle of the temporalis muscle or the auricular region. Patients with masseter PGM often experience functional pain, particularly when chewing hard foods, along with fatigue when chewing and even speaking. Other symptoms include:
    - Limitation of mouth opening, especially if the PGMs are bilateral.
    - Mandibular deflection in unilateral cases.
    - Less frequent symptoms such as sensation of stuffy ear, tinnitus and otalgia.
- Activation mechanisms: The mechanisms of PGM activation in the masseter can be direct or indirect (67, 68):
  - Direct mechanisms:
    - Habitual unilateral chewing.
    - Bruxism (teeth grinding, both day and night).

- Parafunctional habits such as unconscious biting of objects or nails.
- Prolonged dental interventions.
- Overload when chewing hard foods such as nuts.
- Psychological stress.

- Indirect mechanisms:
  - Primary and secondary headaches.
  - Degenerative disorders of the TMJ (arthritis, osteoarthritis).
  - Trigeminal neuropathies (trigeminal neuralgia, atypical odontalgia).
  - Dental and gingival pathologies.
  - Dysfunction of the condyle-disc complex.
  - Cervical musculoskeletal disorders.
  - PGM activation in other muscles, such as the sternocleidomastoid (SCM), upper trapezius, suboccipital, buccinator, pterygoid and temporalis muscles.

- Dry needling: The puncture is performed with the patient in lateral or supine decubitus, with the head turned contralaterally. The therapist palpates the muscle and makes a perpendicular puncture with the needle (0.16 mm x 25 mm), looking for bone contact to fully explore the muscle. In patients with masseter hypertrophy, a 0.25 mm x 40 mm needle may be necessary (67, 68).

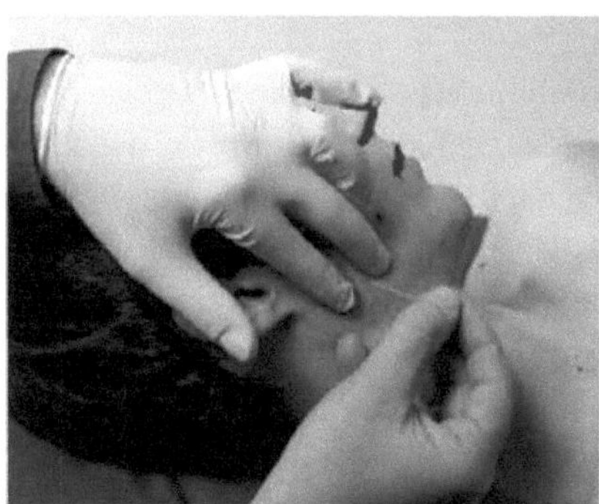

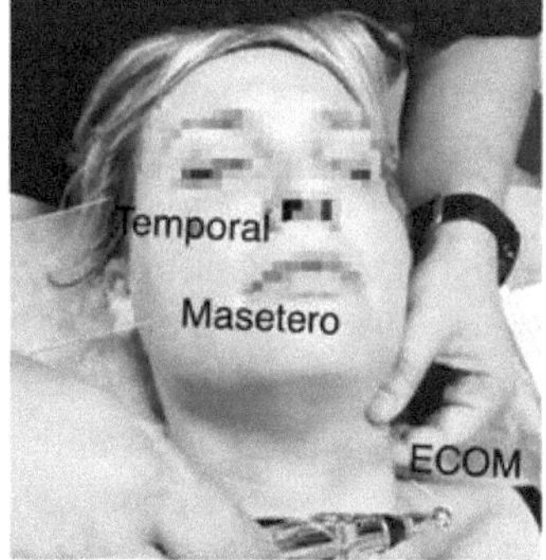

Figure 1. PS in PGM for Masseter (66).

- Hazards and precautions: The masseteric neurovascular bundle lies anterior to the TMJ and posterior to the temporalis tendon, so precautions should be taken to avoid accidental puncture. The facial nerves (temporofacial and cervicofacial) are located close to the superficial fascicle of the masseter. In case of contact with a nerve, the patient may feel a superficial electrical sensation in the face. If this occurs, the needle should be withdrawn and insertion should be restarted at another point nearby (67, 68).

4.1.2. Temporary.

- Trigger points and referred pain: Myofascial trigger points (MTrPs) in the temporalis muscle are easily palpable. The most common referred pain pattern described by Simons et al. encompasses the temporal region, the supraorbital rim (including the eyebrow), the back of the eye, the temporomandibular joint (TMJ), and all maxillary teeth from molars to incisors. The authors of the chapter also mention a variant of referred pain in the posterior portion of the muscle, which includes pain behind the ear and in the mastoid region, without sensation of otalgia. Although PGMs in the temporalis muscle do not usually cause significant limitation of mouth opening, it is common for them to affect mandibular protrusive movement. Pain may be present at rest and increase during mastication, especially when swallowing hard foods (69, 70).
- Clinical symptoms: pain in the temporal region, odontalgia not related to dental problems, restriction of mandibular protrusion movement, exacerbation of pain during mastication on the affected side, pain at rest (69, 70).
- Activation mechanisms: Temporal muscle PGMs can be activated by direct factors such as bruxism (day or night) and muscle overloads caused by dysfunctional chewing habits, especially unilateral chewing. Indirect mechanisms include degenerative or inflammatory TMJ disorders, joint disc dislocations, neuropathic pain (such as auriculotemporal nerve neuralgia), mandibular trauma, craniocervical postural disturbances, upper cervical region problems, and some primary and secondary headaches. In addition, PGMs of the temporalis muscle can be activated as satellites of trigger points in other related muscles, such as the upper trapezius fibers, the sternocleidomastoid (SCM), the suboccipital group, the masseter, and the medial and lateral pterygoids (69, 70).
- Dry needling: To treat PGMs, the patient should be in a lateral or supine position, with the head and neck in a neutral and relaxed

position. Tight bands in the temporalis muscle are usually not easily palpable. It is important to avoid puncturing blood vessels, especially the superficial temporal artery in the anterior portion of the muscle. The needle (0.25 mm x 13 mm) is inserted perpendicularly until it contacts the bone, but very superficially (69, 70).

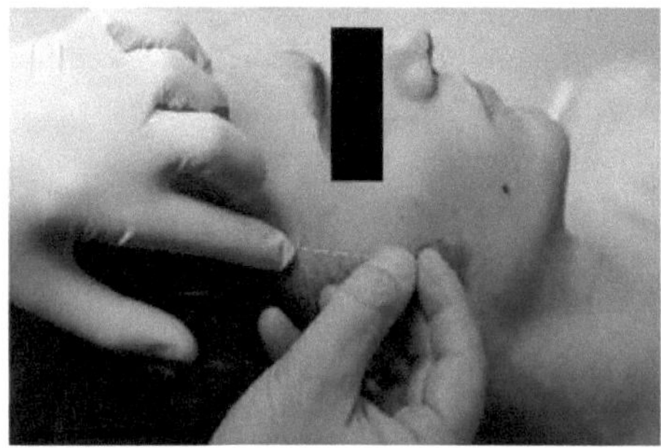
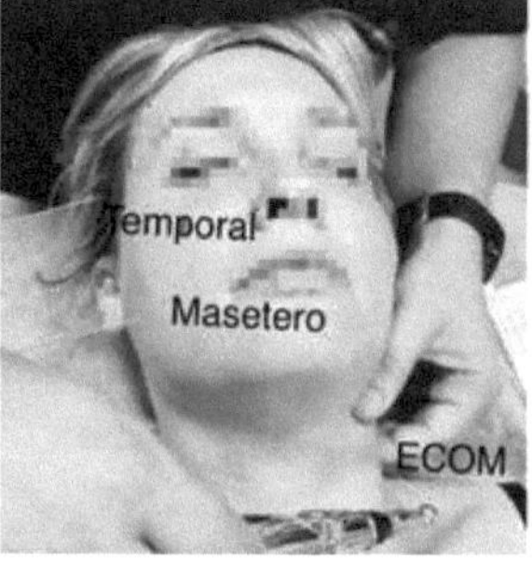

Figure 2. PS for PGM in temporal (66).

- Precautions: Due to the rich innervation of the skin, fascia and temporalis muscle, and the superficial presence of the auriculotemporal nerve, special care should be taken to avoid contact with these nerves during the procedure. In addition, adequate asepsis must be ensured in the scalp area due to its difficulty to disinfect properly (69, 70).

4.1.3. Medial pterygoid.

- Trigger points and referred pain: The medial pterygoid muscle is not easy to palpate, except at its insertion near the angle of the mandible. Although it is possible to access the myofascial trigger points (MTrPs) of this muscle by intraoral palpation, this may cause nausea in some patients, making it difficult to explore. The most common referred pain pattern, according to Simons et al. includes pain in the back of the mouth, pharynx, TMJ (particularly in the posterior pole) and both superficial and deep ear pain (71, 72).
- Symptoms: Patients with PGM of the medial pterygoid usually experience mild limitation of jaw opening, accompanied by contralateral deviation in the last degrees of opening. They may also present with pain when chewing bilaterally or when clenching the teeth in the intercuspal position. In addition, it is common to find pain and restriction laterally to the opposite side when the patient

attempts to move the mandible laterally. Other symptoms include fatigue when chewing, mild dysphagia (difficulty swallowing) and mild pain when swallowing. In some cases, PGMs may generate the sensation of a blocked ear (baro-hypoacusis) (71, 72).

- Activation mechanisms: Direct factors that can activate the medial pterygoid PGMs include surgical trauma, especially after wisdom tooth extraction, prolonged dental interventions that require keeping the mouth open, and parafunctional habits such as bruxism. In addition, muscular overload caused by inadequate masticatory habits is also a triggering factor. Indirect mechanisms include degenerative disorders of the TMJ, problems in the suprahyoid and infrahyoid musculature, dental and mucogingival pathologies, and craniofacial trauma, such as those derived from orthognathic surgeries. This muscle can also activate PGMs in other related muscles, such as the masseter, lateral pterygoid and temporalis (71, 72).
- Dry puncture: Dry puncture of the medial pterygoid muscle can be performed extraorally or intraorally, the former being the most recommended. During the procedure, the patient should keep the jaw open in a submaximal position, using a device that facilitates this position, such as a mouth-opening cue. It is necessary to establish a non-verbal communication system between the patient and the therapist so that the patient can express any discomfort. For the puncture, anatomical landmarks such as the zygomatic arch, mandibular condyle, coronoid process and mandibular notch are located and a needle (0.30 mm x 75 mm) is inserted near the edge of the notch, obliquely downward and medially (71, 72).

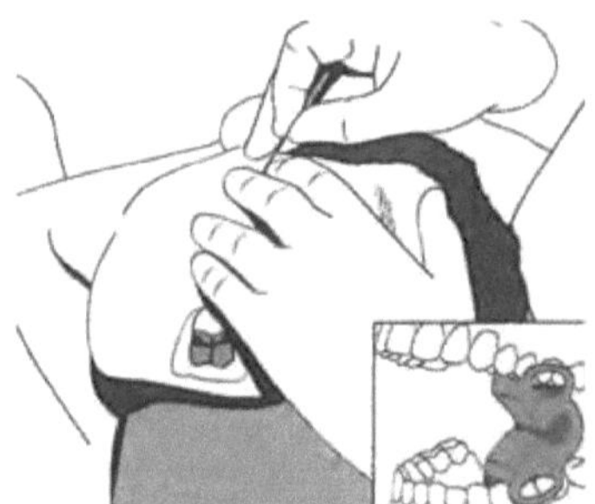
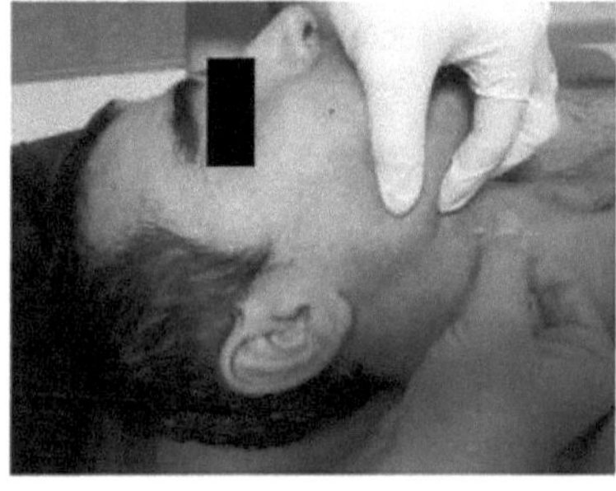

PS for PGM in medial pterygoid (40, 66).

- Precautions: The risk of injuring nearby nerve structures, such as the lingual nerve or branches of the mandibular nerve, is considerable, so appropriate precautions should be taken. There is also a risk of perforating vessels such as the pterygoid artery or plexus. It is important to follow safety and asepsis norms to avoid complications (71, 72).

4.1.4. Lateral pterygoid.

- Trigger points and referred pain of the lateral pterygoid muscle: Myofascial trigger points (MTPs) of the lateral pterygoid muscle are difficult to access due to their deep location, especially in the inferior fibers of the lower division. Intraoral palpation of these MTrPs can cause considerable pain, complicating direct manual treatments. However, dry needling (DP) is the treatment of choice in these cases, provided there are no contraindications (71, 72).
- Referred pain and symptoms: The usual referred pain pattern, described by Simons et al. includes pain in the maxillary region and in the temporomandibular joint (TMJ), sometimes mimicking the characteristic pain of arthritis in this joint. Functional symptoms are usually unilateral and may cause alterations in motor control of the jaw, such as deviation during opening (with a zigzag movement), which is predominantly tilted to the side opposite to the affected muscle. Other symptoms include: Painful limitation of mouth opening and laterotrusion to the opposite side, TMJ joint clicking which sometimes disappears after effective treatment of PGMs, tinnitus (ringing in the ears) may also be a related symptom (71, 72).
- Activation mechanisms: The most common direct mechanisms of PGM activation include parafunctional disorders such as bruxism (day or night) and muscle overload caused by dysfunctional chewing habits, especially unilateral chewing. Alterations of the condyle-disc complex should also be considered. Indirect mechanisms are similar to those affecting the masseter, temporalis and medial pterygoid muscles. In addition, the lateral pterygoid PGMs may be activated as satellites of the masseter, buccinator, medial pterygoid and temporalis PGMs (71, 72).
- Related muscles: masseter, medial pterygoid, buccinator, temporalis (71, 72).

- Dry needling: It is advisable to evaluate and, if necessary, treat the masseter and temporalis muscles first before approaching the puncture of the lateral pterygoid. The PS is performed in a triangular space between the condyle and the mandibular neck, the zygomatic arch and the mandibular notch. The patient should be in lateral or supine decubitus, with the head turned to the opposite side, and it is not necessary to force the mandibular opening, as the puncture can be performed with the mouth closed or ajar. This also facilitates the patient's verbal communication during the procedure. Bone landmarks such as the condyle and zygomatic arch are located, and a 0.25 mm x 40 mm needle is inserted perpendicularly, keeping it close to the zygomatic arch to avoid colliding with the mandibular notch. The needle can be oriented in different directions (anterior, posterior, caudal or cranial) to palpate the muscle for its PGMs (71, 72).

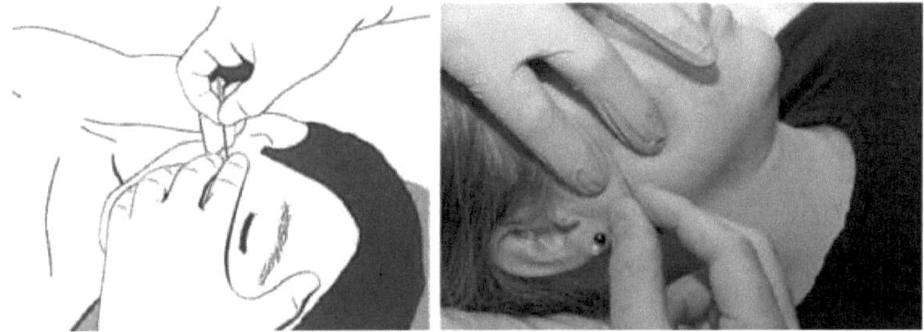

PS in PGM for the lateral pterygoid muscle (40, 66).

- Precautions: Puncture of the lateral pterygoid crosses the deep fascicle of the masseter, so the same precautions should be taken as for this muscle. Since the lateral pterygoid is innervated by multiple nerve branches, the usual precautions should be followed when performing the puncture to avoid complications (71, 72).

4.1.5. Digastric.

- Referred pain and symptoms (73):
    - Posterior belly: The pain referred by myofascial trigger points (MTrPs) in this area projects towards the mastoid process, including the proximal part of the sternocleidomastoid muscle (SCM). Pain may also be referred to the ear. Palpation of the posterior belly is difficult due to its depth and the presence of

neurovascular structures, which may lead to false positives in the diagnosis.

- Anterior belly: PGMs in the anterior belly can cause non-odontogenic odontalgia in the four lower incisors, sometimes accompanied by pain in the middle and anterior part of the tongue. In addition to painful symptoms, PGMs can cause dysfunction of hyo-lingual motor control, with signs of mild dysphagia and alterations in mouth opening rhythm, especially when PGMs are unilateral. Patients often complain of excessive tension in the anterior neck.

- Clinical (73):
  - Anterior belly: Non odontogenic odontalgia in the lower incisors and mild signs of motor dysphagia.
  - Posterior belly: Pain in the proximal part of the ECM and possible referred otalgia.
- Activation mechanisms: PGMs in the digastric muscle are usually activated as satellites of the masticatory or cervical muscles, particularly the ECM. Predisposing factors include dysfunctional craniocervical postures during mastication, swallowing or phonation, as well as alterations of the condyle-disc complex that generate an anomalous unilateral activation pattern, which can activate the digastric PGMs (73).
- Related muscles: Masticatory and cervical muscles.
- Dry needling:
  - Anterior belly: It is performed with the patient in the supine position with a slight craniocervical extension to facilitate access. A 0.25 mm x 25 mm needle is used (73).

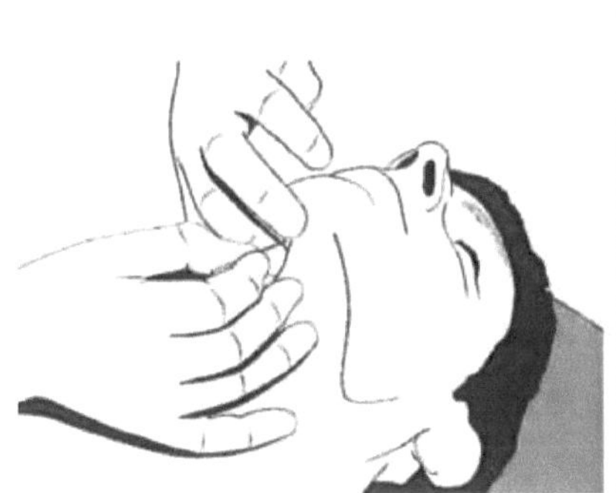

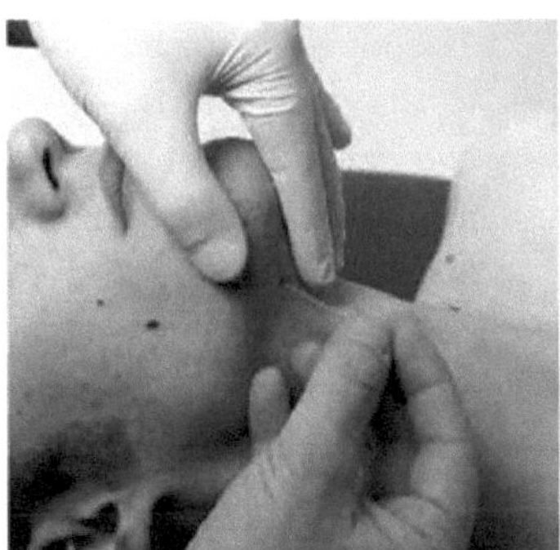

PS for PGM in the anterior belly of the digastric muscle (40, 66).

- Posterior belly: For the puncture, the PGMs are located behind and medial to the angle of the mandible. The physical therapist forceps the PGM with the index and middle fingers, bringing it close to the skin with firm pressure. A 0.16 mm x 25 mm needle is used, with caution due to the risk of damaging nearby neurovascular structures (73).

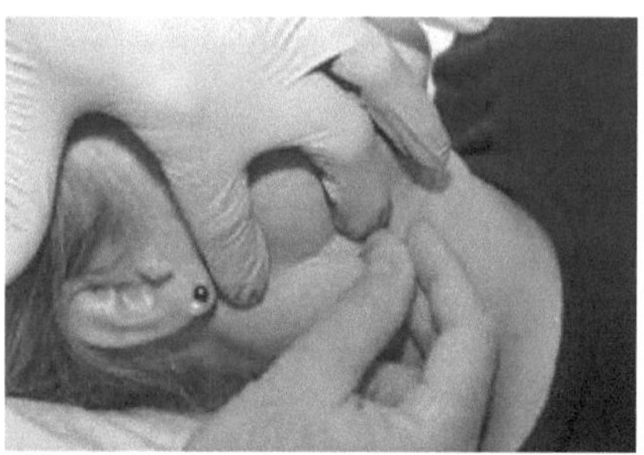

PS for PGM in the posterior belly of the digastric muscle (66).

- Precautions: In the posterior belly, the proximity of neurovascular structures makes it necessary to take precautions to avoid complications. These are similar to the precautions taken in the puncture of the anterior abdomen (73).

4.1.6. Fascial muscles.

- Referred pain and symptoms (74):
  - Major zygomatic muscle: The referred pain pattern described by extends along the edge of the nose, up over the bridge of the nose to the middle of the forehead. PGMs in this muscle may cause muscle tightness when opening the mouth and mild resistance to maintain lip closure.
  - Buccinator muscle: The referred pain projects through the cheek in the maxillary area. It can also generate non-odontogenic odontalgia in the canines and incisors of the maxillary area. Other symptoms include masticatory fatigue and mild pain when chewing on the affected side.

- Procero muscle: PGMs may report deep pain in the central part of the nasal bone and the upper part of the nasal cartilages, even inside the nasal cavity. The pain may be described as similar to that caused by sinusitis, extending to the sides of the nose.
- Corrugator muscle of the eyebrow: The referred pain is slightly above the middle part of the ocular orbit, extending towards the inner corner of the eye and the nasal cartilage.

- Clinical (74):
  - Major zygomatic muscle: Tension when opening the mouth and slight difficulty in maintaining lip closure.
  - Buccinator muscle: masticatory fatigue and pain during mastication, non-odontogenic odontalgia.
  - Procero and corrugator muscles of the eyebrow: Deep facial pain similar to sinusitis, ocular pain.
- Activation mechanisms (74):
  - Greater zygomatic and buccinator: PGMs are usually activated as secondary to those of the masticatory musculature.
  - Procero and brow corrugator: PGMs are activated by sustained facial gestures such as frowning, headaches with photophobia, eye strain or astigmatism.
- Related muscles: Masticatory muscles.
- Dry needling:
  - Buccinator muscle: The patient should be in supine or lateral decubitus. The PGMs are located in the middle part of the cheek, equidistant between the angle of the mouth and the mandibular ramus. The muscle is palpated in clamp with one finger inside the mouth and the other outside. The needle is inserted towards the internal finger, taking care not to accidentally puncture it (74).
  - Zygomaticus major muscle: The puncture is similar to that of the buccinator, but in a higher area, near the edge of the nose (74).

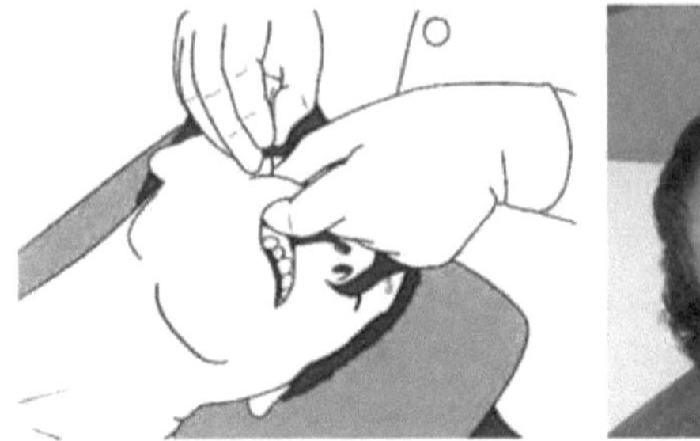
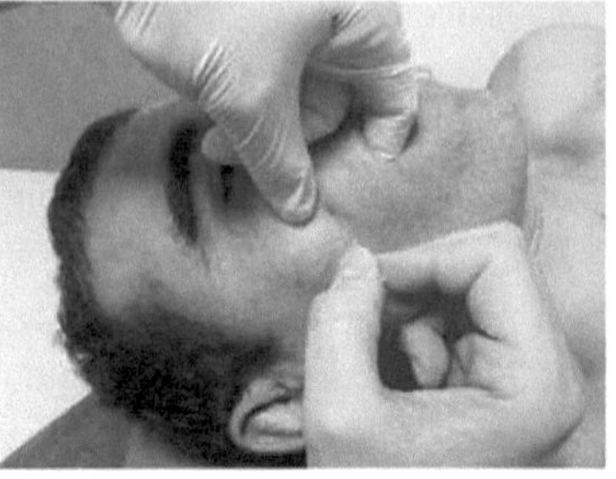

PS for PGM in zygomatic major (40, 66).

- Procero and corrugator muscles of the eyebrow: These muscles can be clamped flat or in clamp. The twisting technique is recommended for these muscles (74).

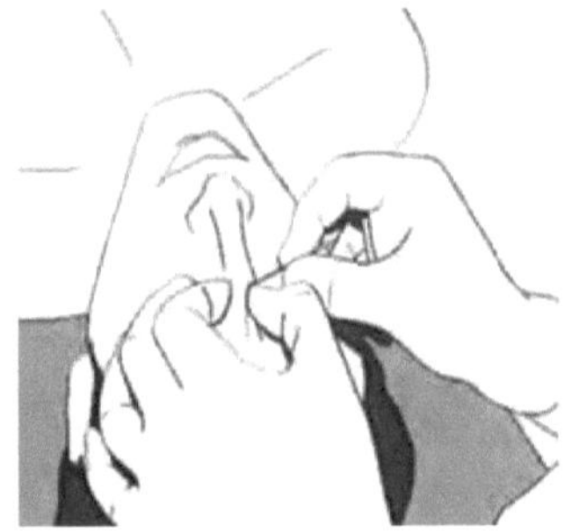
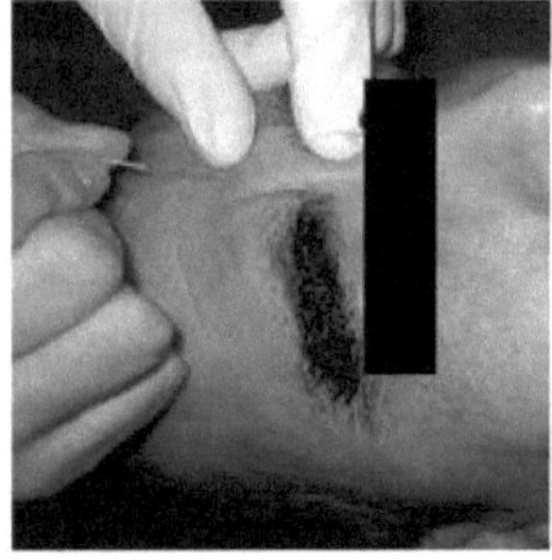

PS for PGM in procero with clamp technique (40, 66).

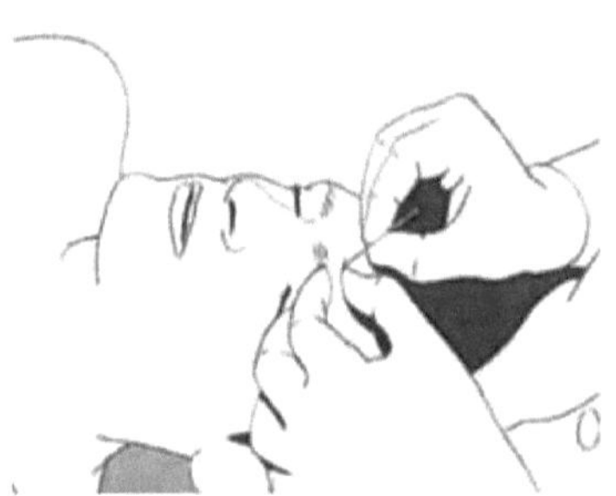
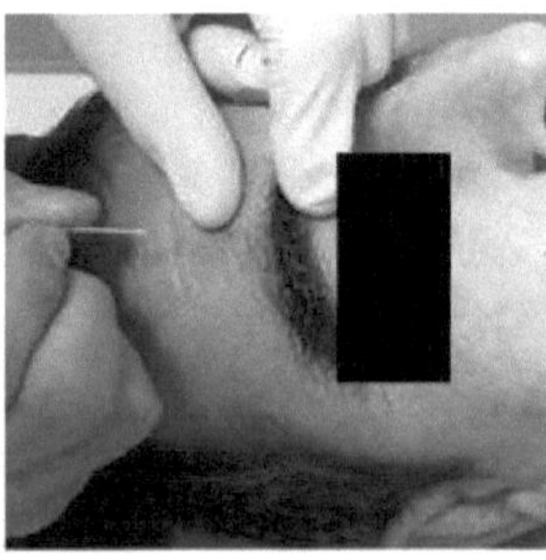

Figure 9. PS for PGM in corrugator of the eyebrow (40, 66).

- A 0.16 mm x 25 mm needle is recommended for all these muscles.

- Dangers and precautions: For the buccinator and zygomaticus major muscles, it is important to be careful with nearby nerve structures (74).

4.2. Musculature of the neck.

4.2.1. Trapeze.

- Activation mechanisms (75, 76):
  - Direct: Cervical trauma, repetitive actions (swimming, using the telephone), inadequate postures (computer work without ergonomics).
  - Indirect: Dysfunction of other muscles and visceral pathologies (liver diseases, ulcers).
- Effects on mobility: increased muscle tension, but without severe restriction of mobility. Painful movements: contralateral tilt, shoulder abduction.
- Diagnosis and differential tests: Compression test to differentiate between PGM of the trapezius and other muscles.
- Hazards and precautions (75, 76):
  - Upper Trapezius, PGM1: The spinal nerve enters the trapezius, dividing into a plexus that receives contributions from C2-C4. The anterior border of the trapezius is full of nerve branches, which can cause pain during puncture. It is essential to palpate the nerve to avoid accidental punctures and to observe the patient's reaction. The forceps technique during puncture reduces the risk of pneumothorax.
  - Lower Trapezius, PGM4: The medial border of the scapula should be palpated to ensure that it is between the needle and the rib cage. The PGM is usually in a safe area over the scapula, but if this is not the case, the PGM3 technique will be applied.

Main PGMs for trapezius (75, 76):

- PGM 1 (Upper trapezius, clavicular portion):
  - Location: Middle part of the anterior border.
  - Referred pain: Towards the posterior part of the pinna, temples and masseter region.
  - Secondary activation: Can activate PGMs in the ECM and masseter.
  - Dry needling:

- Position: Patient in prone position.
- Needle: 0.25 mm x 25 mm, clamp and ventral direction of the needle.
- Effects: Local spasms.

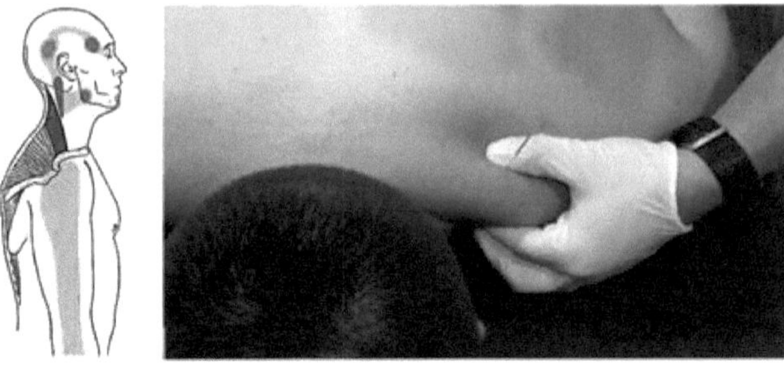

Referred pain from the PGMs (gray area and dots in the figure) of the clavicular fibers of the upper trapezius towards the arm (PGM1) and puncture (PGM1) of the upper trapezius in the most anterior portion (40).

- PGM2 (Upper trapezius, acromial portion):
  - Referred pain: Towards the suboccipital region.
  - Effects: Increased tension and thickness of the affected muscle.
  - PS:
    - Position: Prone position.
    - Needle: 0.30 mm x 40 mm, ventral direction.

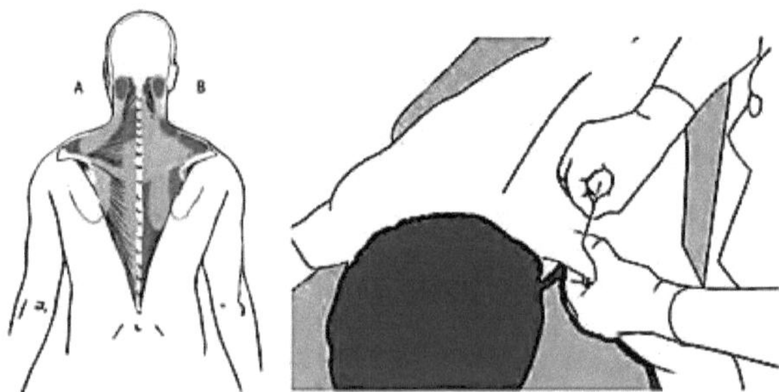

Figure 2. A. Referred pain pattern of the posterior fibers of the upper trapezius (PGM2). B. Most common referred pain pattern of the central PGMs of the lower trapezius (PGM3). As well as the puncture of the upper trapezius (40).

- PGM 3 (Lower Trapezius):
  - Location: Lower fibers.
  - Referred pain: Deep and unpleasant pain in the upper trapezius; may cause elevation and anterior tilt of the scapula.
  - PS:
    - Position: Prone position with arm in abduction.
    - Needle: 0.25 mm x 25 mm, horizontal direction and tangential to the thorax of the needle accompanied by flat palpation.

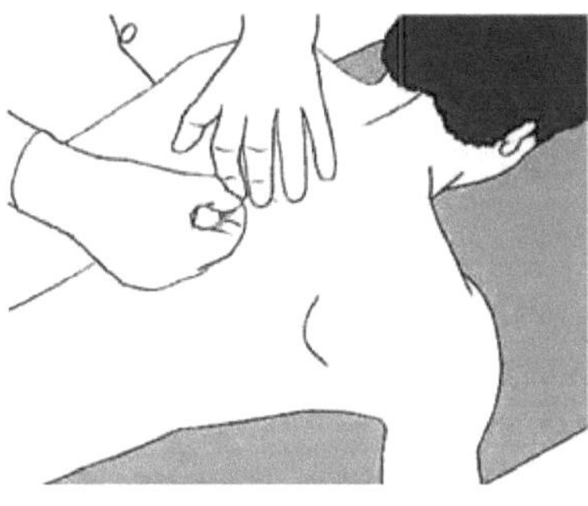
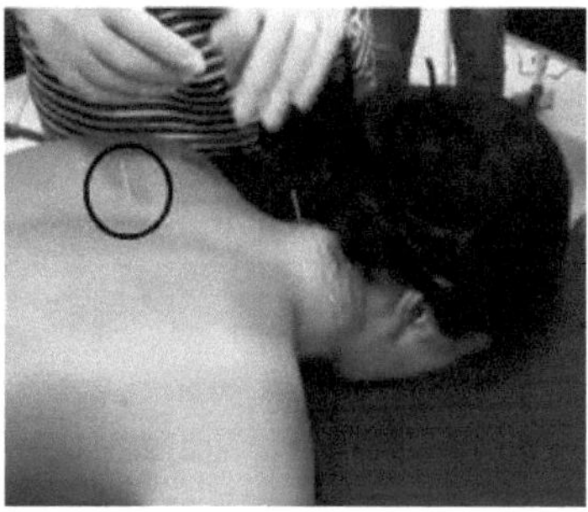

Puncture of the PGMs of the lower trapezius (indicated by a circle in the figure on the right) (40, 66).

- PGM 4 (Insertional):
  - Location: Spine of the scapula.
  - Symptoms: Constant stinging sensation in the medial border of the scapula.
  - PS:
    - Position: Prone or lateral decubitus with arm in abduction.
    - Needle: 0.25 mm x 25 mm, direction to the spine of the scapula.
- PGM 5 (Middle Trapezius):
  - Location: Central part.
  - Symptoms: May cause piloerection and chills on the lateral aspect of the arm.
  - PS: Similar to PGM3 with needle introduction at an angle to avoid lung injury.
- PGM 6 (Insertional of the middle trapezius):
  - Location: Near the acromion.
  - Referred pain: To this area.
  - PS:

- Position: Prone position.
- Needle: 0.30 mm x 50 mm, oblique direction towards the supraspinous fossa.

- PGM 7 (Cutaneous):
  - Description: Chance finding related to piloerection; rarely requires intervention.
  - Symptoms and Referred Pain:
  - Headaches and cervical pain: Relationship with PGM in the upper trapezius.
  - Carpal tunnel syndrome: Possible correlation.
  - Other symptoms: photophobia in patients with chronic post-traumatic cervical syndrome.
  - PS: Surface technique similar to PGM5.

4.2.2. Sternocleidomastoid.

The sternocleidomastoid muscle (SCM) is prone to develop myofascial trigger points (MTrPs) that can cause symptoms in various areas of the body. MTPs can be located in both the sternal and clavicular portions of the SCM, and each has a distinct pattern of referred pain (77, 78).

- Referred pain (77, 78):
  - Sternal division: Pain may radiate to the vertex of the head, occipital region, cheek, eye and upper sternum. Patients may experience vegetative symptoms, such as excessive tearing, eye redness, blurred vision, sinus congestion, dysphagia ("ball in the throat" sensation), and atypical symptoms such as dry cough or tickle in the throat.
  - Clavicular division: Causes referred pain mainly in the forehead and auricular area, which may include tinnitus or auditory disturbances. In addition, PGMs in this area may cause dizziness, vertigo and spatial perception problems.
- Additional symptoms (77, 78):
  - Dizziness and vertigo: ECM PGMs can cause a feeling of disorientation or lightheadedness, often described as a "bobbing in the head" sensation, which is less common than traditional vertigo.

- Mobility restriction: Unlike other cervical muscles, the PGMs in the ECM do not usually severely restrict neck movement.
- Nausea and vomiting: In some cases, dizziness may also be accompanied by these symptoms.

- ECM PGMs can be activated by several factors (77, 78):
    - Postural: Keeping the head in a forward, rotated or extended position for a long time can trigger PGMs.
    - Traumatic: Whiplash, common in traffic accidents, is a frequent triggering factor for PGMs in the ECM.
    - Respiratory: Patients with respiratory diseases such as asthma or chronic obstructive pulmonary disease (COPD) may overuse the ECM, which contributes to the formation of PGMs.
    - Indirect factors: PGMs in other muscles such as the pectoralis major, scalenes or digastric may activate the PGMs of the ECM.
- Dry needling of the ECM: Dry needling is a treatment that can be effective in deactivating ECM PGMs. However, there are associated risks due to the proximity of important structures such as the external jugular vein and accessory spinal nerve. It is crucial that the therapist follows specific precautions to avoid complications such as ecchymosis or nerve damage. The technique involves careful palpation of the muscle and applying the needle at a safe angle to avoid underlying structures (77, 78).

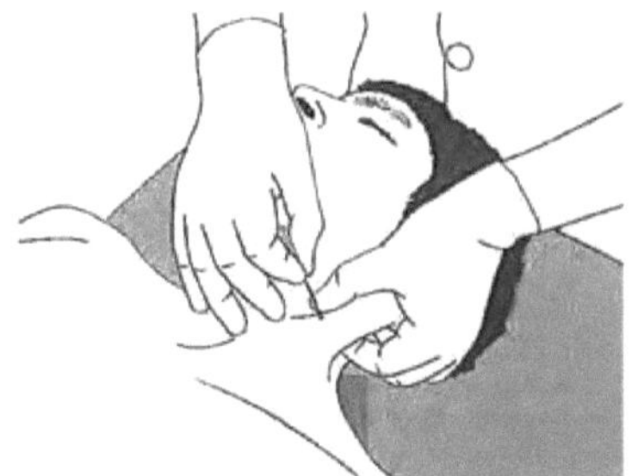
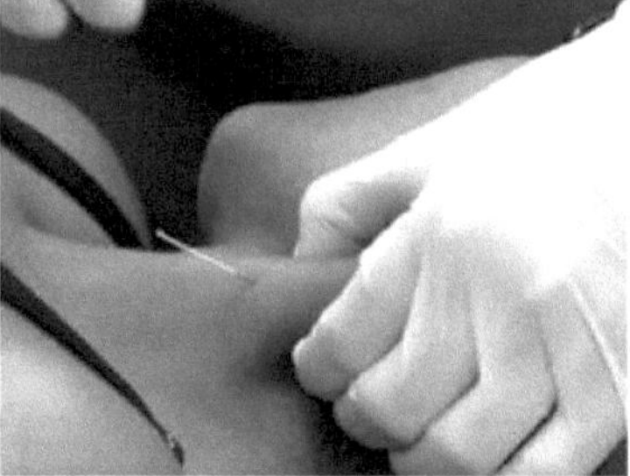

Figure 7. Dry puncture of the PGMs of the ECM muscle (40, 66).

- Precautions: It is important to avoid deep puncture in the lower area of the clavicular portion of the ECM, as it is close to the pulmonary apex and there may be a risk of pneumothorax if punctured too deep (77, 78).

4.2.3. Scalenes.

Myofascial trigger points (MTPs) in the scalene muscles can generate referred pain in different areas, both in the cervico-scapular region and in the upper limb. Pain may also radiate to the head, anterior thorax or upper dorsal area, which may be confused with visceral or radicular pathologies (79, 80).

- Referred pain and symptoms (79, 80):
    - Cervical and shoulder: Pain may be localized in the region of the upper trapezius, anterior shoulder, biceps, triceps and radial part of the forearm, reaching the thumb and index finger. This pain may simulate involvement of the C5-C6 nerve roots.
    - Anterior chest: On the left side, pain may be confused with respiratory or cardiac problems. Other muscles, such as the pectoralis major or intercostal muscles, should also be evaluated for possible secondary trigger point activation.
    - Dorsal region and scapula: The scalenes can cause pain in the upper scapula and interscapular region, which could be mistaken for problems in the rhomboid or levator scapulae.
    - Pain related to movements: Upper limb elevation movements or breathing (coughing, sneezing, deep breathing) may exacerbate pain. Relief can be obtained by passively elevating the arm or by the "scalene relief test".
- Scalene PGMs can be activated by a variety of factors (79, 80):
    - Cervical trauma.
    - Activities involving heavy loads or repetitive movements.
    - Respiratory pathologies that increase the use of upper thoracic breathing.
    - Inadequate posture, especially during work or daily activities.
    - Dysmetry of the lower limbs, scoliosis, or small hemipelvis that forces the scalenes to compensate for the inclination of the cervical spine.
    - The scalenes may also be associated with thoracic gorge syndrome (TDS), due to their involvement in the elevation of the first rib, which may compress the brachial plexus.

- Superficial dry needling is highly effective for the scalenes. In case of deep puncture (79, 80):
  - Anterior scalene: The patient should be in lateral decubitus. The muscle is located by palpating under the clavicle and the needle is inserted obliquely, avoiding vasculonervous structures.
  - Middle scalene: A similar approach to the anterior scalene is used, with a deeper, posteriorly oriented insertion to avoid the brachial plexus.
  - Due to the risk of lung damage, deep dry needling of the posterior scalene is not recommended.

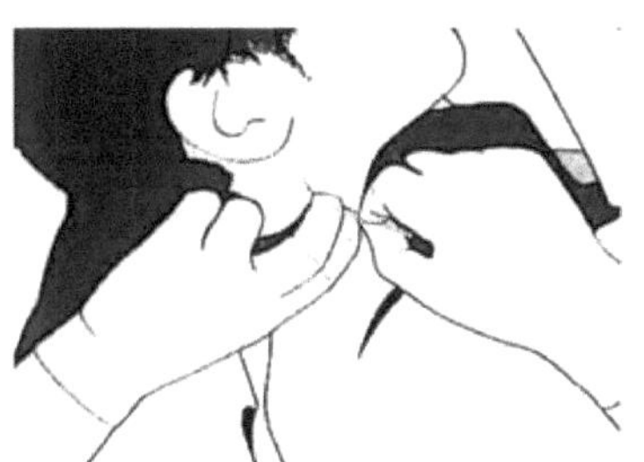

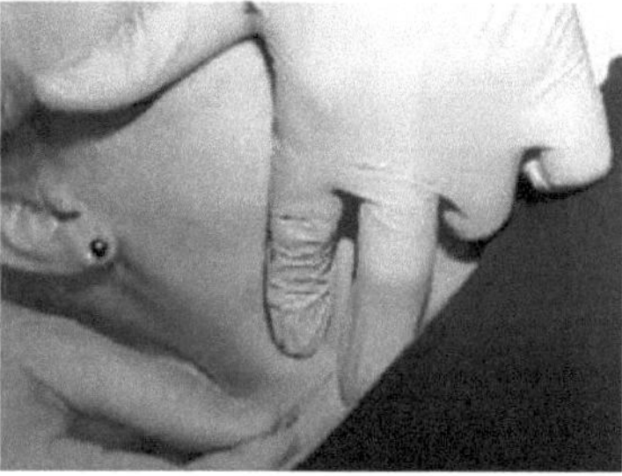

Figure 8. Dry puncture of the anterior scalene and middle scalene (40, 66).

- Precautions: When performing PS on the scalenes, accidental puncture of the external jugular vein, subclavian artery, and pulmonary apex should be avoided. In addition, caution with the brachial plexus and other nearby sensitive structures is crucial. This array of symptoms and triggering mechanisms requires careful clinical evaluation for appropriate treatment (79, 80).

4.2.4. Splenium.

- PGM localization and palpation: The trigger points of the splenius of the head are found by palpation on the medial aspect of the muscle, where it attaches to the superior border of the trapezius. This muscle can be palpated in a triangle bounded by the ECM anteriorly, the upper trapezius fibers posteriorly, and the levator scapulae inferiorly. The splenius fibers are distinguished by their diagonal orientation and by being activated during homolateral rotation of the head, unlike the ECM and upper trapezius, which are contralateral rotators. To palpate the PGMs of the splenius of the head, it is recommended to place the cervical region in slight flexion and contralateral rotation, which facilitates identification of the taut bands. However, in some cases, the muscle may be sufficiently tight to be palpable even in a neutral position, such as prone. This position makes it possible to evaluate both splenii of the head and detect differences in tissue texture prior to a more specific examination (81, 82).

- Referred pain: The splenium of the head presents a pattern of referred pain, commonly associated with headaches homolateral to the vertex. However, clinical experience shows a broader pattern that includes headaches in the suboccipital, occipital, frontal, ocular and ear regions, as well as tinnitus. For the splenium of the neck, there are two PGM zones. The first is located in the central region of the muscle, between the upper trapezius and levator scapulae, at the level of the spinous process of C7. Palpation at this level is also performed with the cervical spine in slight flexion and contralateral rotation, and symptoms usually include neck angle pain and cervical stiffness, which are aggravated by homolateral cervical rotation. The second PGM zone is located at the insertion of the splenius of the neck into the posterior tubercles of the upper cervical vertebrae. Here, deep palpation can elicit characteristic pain toward the occipital region and posterior orbit. Although the overlap of muscles in this area makes it difficult to determine with certainty the source of pain, it is not crucial in clinical practice (81, 82).
- Functional limitations: PGMs of the splenius of the head and neck often limit passive contralateral flexion and rotation, as well as active homolateral rotation of the head and neck. These dysfunctions are frequently associated with joint problems in the cervical and upper thoracic region, sharing referred pain patterns.
- Activation mechanisms: The two most common mechanisms that activate the PGMs of the splenius muscles are postural stress and whiplash. Sustained and repetitive extensions or rotations of the head, as well as improper postures, can overload these muscles, favoring the development of PGMs. In the case of whiplash, the splenius of the head is one of the most frequently affected muscles (81, 82).
- PS of the splenium of the head (81, 82):
  - Positions:

- Prone decubitus: The patient keeps the head in a neutral position. The physical therapist is positioned at the head of the table, on the opposite side of the muscle to be treated.
- Lateral Decubitus: The head is positioned with the head slightly flexed and rotated to the opposite side, which facilitates the identification and palpation of the muscle.

- Needle: A 0.25 mm x 25 mm needle is used to access the PGMs in the central region of the muscle, which are located at the subcutaneous level.

- PS of the splenium of the neck (81, 82):
  - Position: The patient is in lateral decubitus contralateral to the affected side, with the head supported by a pillow and the cervical spine in neutral position.
  - Puncture: A 0.25 mm x 25 mm needle is used, directing it obliquely medially and slightly posteriorly, in the region just behind the levator scapulae and in front of the anterior border of the upper trapezius.
  - Insertional Points: The technique for puncture of the insertional PGM of the neck splenius is similar to that used for other cervical muscles, such as the neck semispinatus and cervical multifidus.

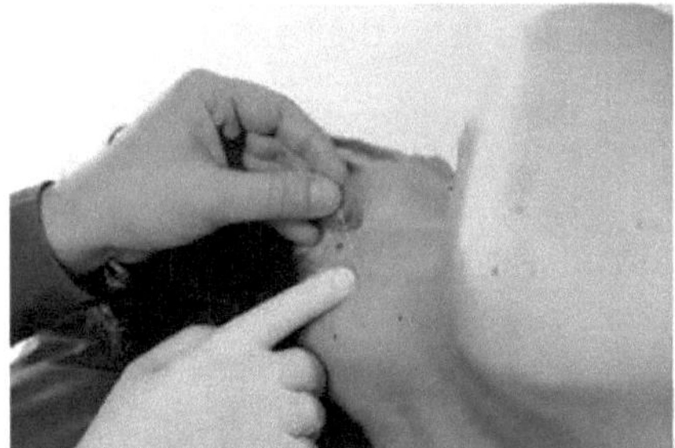

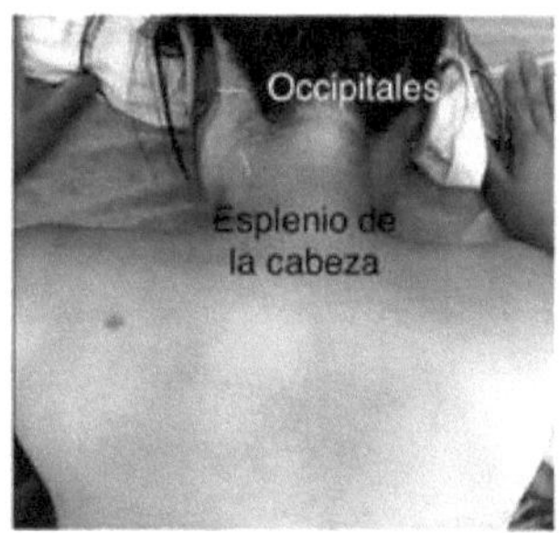

PS for PGM in splenium of the head (66).

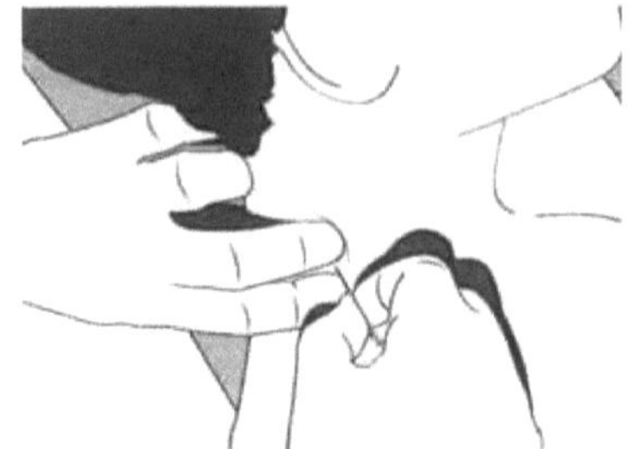 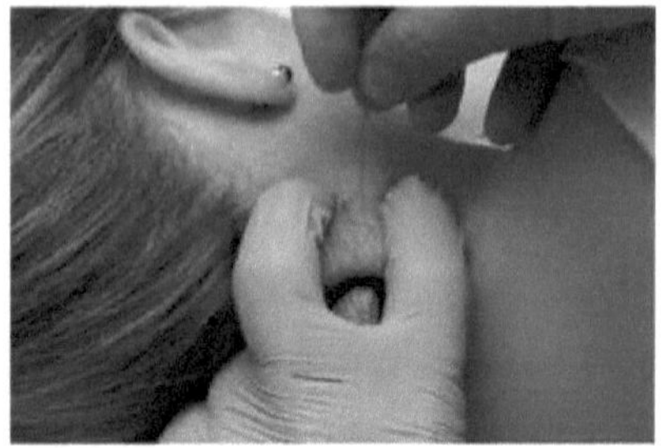

PS for PGM in splenium of the neck (40, 66).

- Hazards and precautions (81, 82):
  - Splenium of the Head: Due to the proximity of the vertebral artery, if deep puncture is performed above C2, the needle should be directed towards the mastoid process to minimize risks.
  - Neck splenium: There is a risk of puncture of the lung. To avoid this, the needle should not be directed caudally, but only medially and slightly posteriorly.

4.2.5. Very long and semi-spiny head.

- PG, referred pain and activation mechanisms (83, 84):
  - Semispinous of the head:
    - Structure: The semispinous muscle of the head is divided into three regions: superior, middle and inferior, which allows the existence of PGMs in each of these divisions.
    - Referred pain patterns:
      - Upper division: PGM localization in the suboccipital area, 1-2 cm from the midline. Referred banded pain extending from the occipital region to the temporal and frontal areas, often mistaken for tension or cervicogenic headache.
      - Middle division: PGM location lateral to the spinous processes of C3-C4. Referred pain in projection to the occipital region on the same side as the PGMs.
      - Inferior division: Localization between C7 and T2. No specific referred pain pattern has been described.
    - Palpation: Difficulty in manual palpation due to coverage by the upper trapezius and splenius of the head. Tight bands can be palpated if the upper trapezius is relaxed.

- Very long of the head (83, 84):
    - Location: From C2 to the junction of C3-C4.
    - Referred pain: Concentrated in the region of the ear, neck and behind the eye.
    - Common Symptoms: Headache following the described pain patterns. Hypersensitivity to pressure in the back of the head and neck. Painful limitation of cervical mobility, especially in flexion. Possible joint dysfunction in the upper cervical region (C0-C3).
    - Activation Mechanisms: Acute trauma (whiplash). Postural stress such as prolonged sitting with the head in a forward position.
    - Activation of other muscles: PGM of adjacent muscles such as upper trapezius and splenius of the head.
    - Radicular pathology or joint dysfunctions: In the cervical spine these can be factors that perpetuate activation.

- PS (83, 84):
  - Technique for head semispinous:
    - Patient Position: Prone decubitus, head in neutral position.
    - Needle: 0.25 mm x 25 mm.
    - Cranial insertion: Directed towards the occipital bone to avoid the vertebral artery.
    - Precautions: Avoid puncture of the greater occipital nerve.
  - Puncture of central PGMs:
    - Needle: 0.25 mm x 25 mm.
    - Direction: Posteroanterior, taking care not to puncture the greater occipital nerve.
    - Risks: Use of needles longer than the recommended length may cause accidental puncture of the vertebral artery, vertebral canal, foramen magnum and zygapophyseal joints.

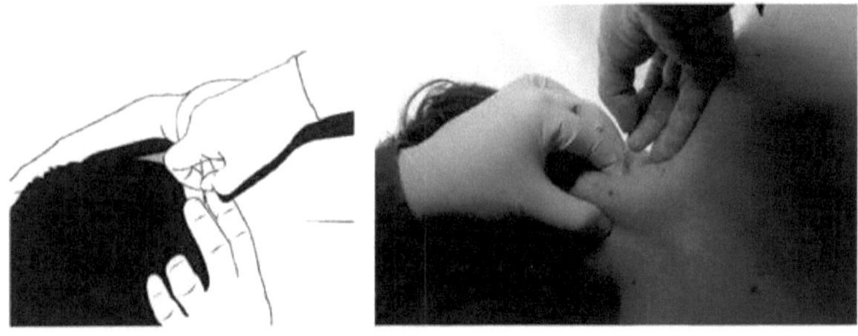

PS for PGM in semispinous of the head and neck (40, 66).

- Technique for head lengthening:
  - Needle: 0.25 mm x 25 mm.
  - Direction: Anterior and lateral, at the height of C3.
  - Caution: Difficult to identify below C4, no significant risks.

4.2.6. Suboccipital.

Myofascial trigger points (MTrPs) in the suboccipital muscles are a common source of referred pain, mainly in the head and cervical region. Due to the depth of these muscles, it is difficult to detect MTrPs by direct palpation. Instead, indicators such as sensitivity to deep pressure and tissue tension in the suboccipital region are used. The occurrence of referred pain on pressure in this area and increased pain on active craniocervical contractions are also key diagnostic criteria (85, 86).

- Referred pain and associated symptoms: PGMs in the suboccipital muscles often cause a pattern of intracranial referred pain that spreads to several areas, including occipital, temporal, frontal, and eye. This type of pain is often confused with other conditions, such as tension headache, cervicogenic headache, occipital neuralgia, or chronic neck pain. In some cases, PGMs in this area may generate bilateral pain, and it is important to note the absence of pain in the suboccipital region itself, which could be associated with PGMs in other nearby muscles (85, 86).
- Several factors can activate PGMs in the suboccipital muscles, including (85, 86):
  - Maintained postures, especially those involving prolonged flexion, extension or rotation of the head, such as forward head position.
  - Uncorrected visual defects that force an unnatural head position.

- Repetitive head movements.
- Whiplash injuries, which frequently cause headaches and dizziness.
- PGMs in the suboccipital muscles are also associated with restricted mobility in the upper cervical spine, especially in flexion, lateral tilt, and craniocervical rotation. In particular, restriction in flexion may be indicative of joint dysfunction at C0-C1 or neural tissue mechanosensitivity.

- Diagnosis and treatment: Diagnosis of PGMs in the suboccipital muscles can be supported by tests such as the Flexion-Rotation Test (FRT), which measures the passive mobility of the cervical spine in rotation. A positive FRT result, indicating less than 33° of rotation, may be indicative of joint dysfunction or muscle shortening, and is a commonly used test to diagnose cervicogenic headache. Treatment of MGPs in this region includes techniques such as dry needling, although it is important to exercise caution when performing this procedure, especially to avoid damage to the vertebral artery or greater occipital nerve. Dry needling is mainly recommended for the inferior oblique muscle of the head due to its accessibility (85, 86).
- PS (85, 86):
  - Patient position: The patient should be in prone decubitus (face down), with the head in neutral position, avoiding any cervical extension. This position allows safer and more direct access to the muscle without compromising adjacent structures.
  - Needle size: It is recommended to use a 0.30 mm x 40 mm needle, suitable for the depth of the inferior oblique muscle.
  - Direction of puncture: The needle should be directed at a posteroanterior and slightly medial angle, aiming towards the lamina of C2, but always avoiding a cranial tilt to minimize risks.

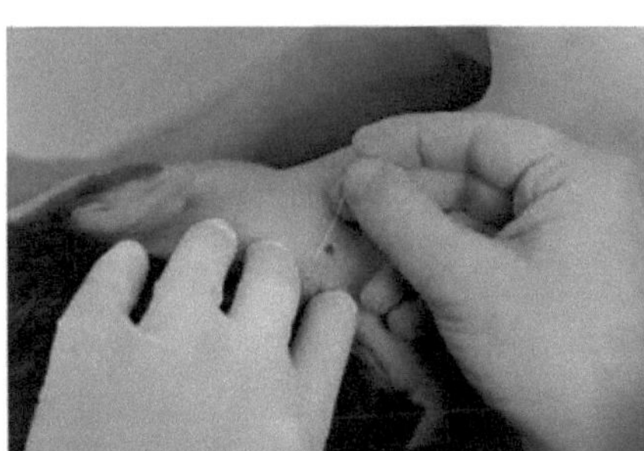

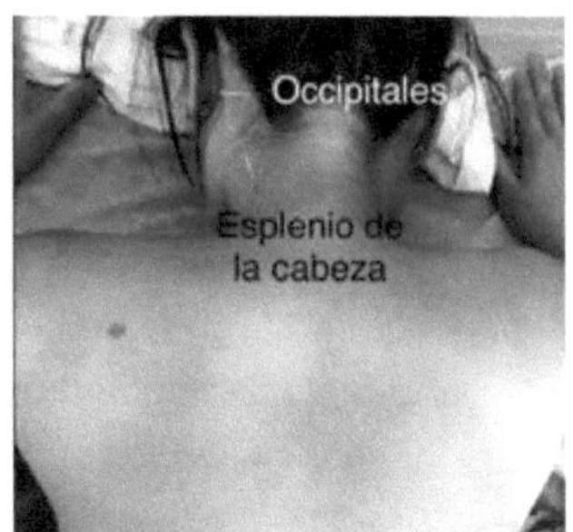

Figure 12. PS in PGM for suboccipital (66).

- Precautions (85, 86):
  - Vertebral artery: It is essential to avoid any cranial orientation of the needle so as not to damage this artery, which is close to the puncture area.
  - Greater occipital nerve: This nerve passes under and in front of the inferior oblique muscle, so care must be taken not to injure it during the puncture.
  - These points ensure safe and effective puncture of the inferior oblique muscle of the head in myofascial trigger point treatments.

4.3. Scapular and shoulder region.

4.3.1. Elevator of the scapula.

- Referred pain and symptoms (87, 88):
  - Neck pain: Localized in the cervical angle with a pattern of irradiation to the medial border of the scapula and posterior shoulder.
  - Limitation of neck mobility: Especially noticeable when stretching or contracting the muscle, resulting in cervical stiffness, evidenced by active homolateral rotation of the neck.
  - Alteration in scapular function: It may affect the scapulohumeral rhythm, predisposing the shoulder to lesions in the subacromial space.
- Trigger mechanisms: PGMs of the levator scapulae can be triggered by postural tension and head forward, use of the telephone between the shoulder and head, psychological stress, overload from prolonged computer work or repetitive neck movements, overstretching or shortening positions, such as sleeping on the stomach (87, 88).
- Related muscles (87, 88):
  - Agonists: neck splenius, middle and posterior scalenes, and rhomboids.
  - Antagonists: Serratus anterior (inferior fibers), lower trapezius and latissimus dorsi. The upper trapezius and sternocleidomastoid frequently present concomitant MGP, the former on the homolateral side and the latter on the contralateral side.
- Dry needling: Percutaneous electrostimulation of the PGMs of the levator scapulae has shown effectiveness in the treatment of pain and

cervical mobility in patients with shoulder and neck pain. The needling procedure will be as follows (87, 88).

- PGM Central:
  - Patient in lateral decubitus on the healthy side.
  - Palpation and clamping of the muscle.
  - Needle insertion 0.30 mm x 40 mm medially and slightly caudal.
- Insertional PGM:
  - Patient in lateral decubitus on the affected side, with the shoulder in 90º flexion, external rotation and retraction.
  - Insertion of a 0.25 mm x 25 mm needle parallel to the thorax, towards the superior angle of the scapula.
- Alternative access for central PGMs covered by trapeze:
  - Similar to the dorsal scapular nerve block approach.
  - Clamp and needle clamp 0.30 mm x 50 mm in cranial and lateral direction.

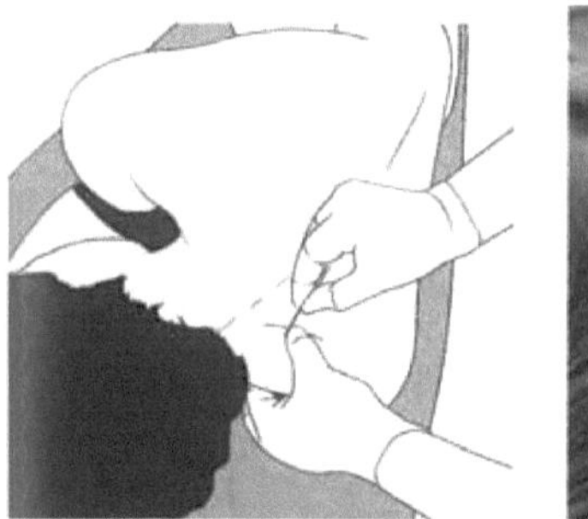
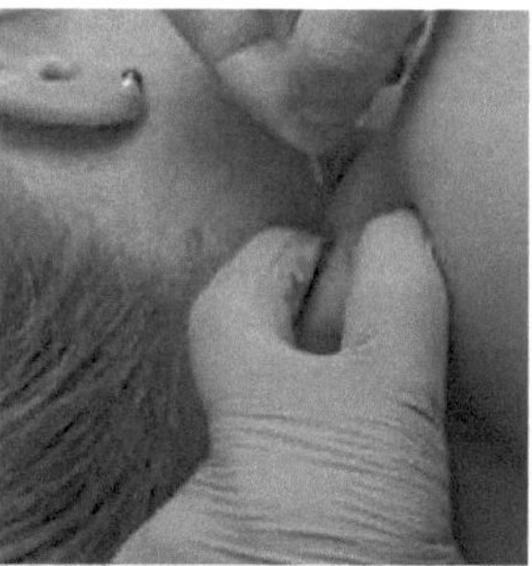

Figure 13. PS in PGM for central of the levator scapulae (40, 66).

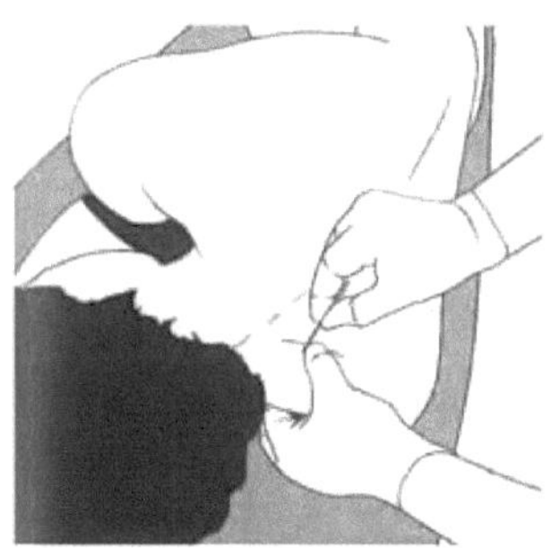
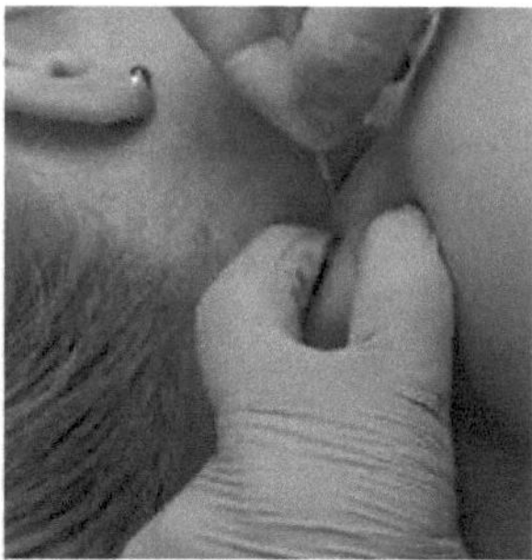

Figure 14. PS in PGM for insertion of the levator scapulae (40, 66).

- Hazards and precautions: There is a risk of pneumothorax during invasive treatment of the levator scapulae, so the use of the clamp approach is recommended whenever possible (87, 88).

4.3.2. Infraspinatus.

- Trigger points and referred pain: The infraspinatus muscle is one of the main causes of referred pain to the shoulder joint, together with the supraspinatus and, sometimes, the levator scapulae. Bron et al. demonstrated that infraspinatus trigger points (TGP) are the most prevalent in patients with chronic non-traumatic shoulder pain, frequently occurring in its fibers. This pain tends to be located in the anterior aspect of the shoulder joint, extending to the anterolateral aspect of the arm, the forearm and the radial border of the hand, and may radiate to the fingers and the posterosuperior cervical region (89, 90).
- Patients often experience associated symptoms such as (89, 90):
  - Difficulty in activities that combine adduction and internal rotation (e.g., fastening a bra, taking out a wallet).
  - Feeling of heaviness and weakness.
  - Paresthesias such as burning or tingling in the homolateral upper limb.
  - Fatigue of the shoulder girdle, weakness of grip and hyperhidrosis in the affected area.
  - Shoulder instability associated with weakness in contraction during external rotation.
- PGM location: The infraspinatus PGMs are typically found in the medial third of the muscle, although they are often closer to the medial third. Simons et al. have documented an insertional PGM at the medial border of the scapula (89, 90).
- Related muscles (89, 90):
  - Agonists: teres minor, posterior deltoid (shoulder external rotation), and other rotator cuff muscles (shoulder stability).
  - Antagonists: subscapularis, pectoralis major and anterior deltoid.
- PS can be performed in different positions: Lateral decubitus on the healthy side, with the shoulder in 70°-90° of flexion. Prone decubitus, with the arm along the body or outside the edge of the stretcher. Procedure (89, 90):

- Lateral decubitus: The patient is positioned on the healthy side, the shoulder in flexion position, and the forearm supported. A 0.30 mm x 40 mm needle is introduced towards the scapula.
- Prone decubitus: The patient can be with the arm along the body or extended.

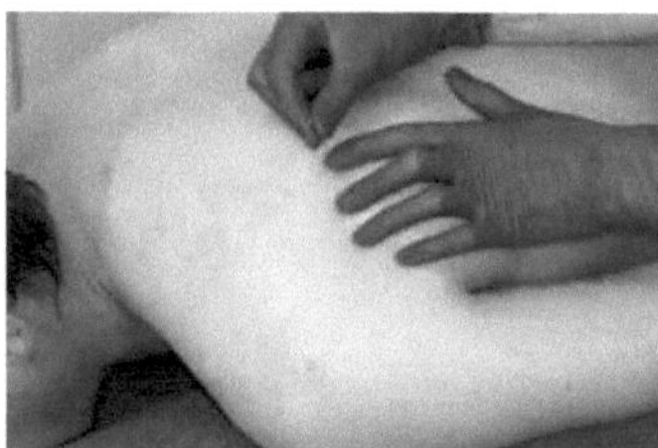
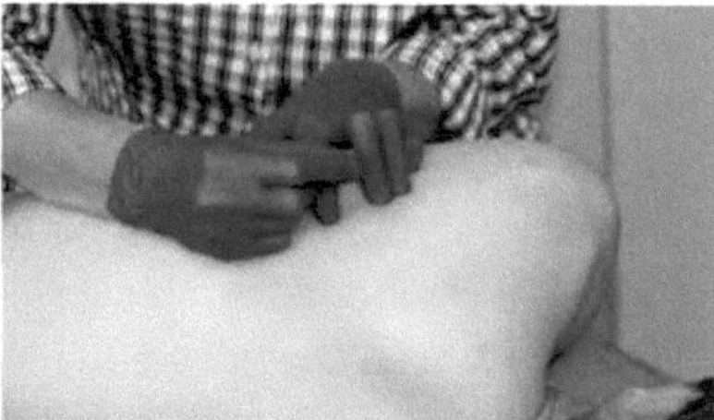

PS for PGM in infraspinatus in posterior decubitus and lateral decubitus (66).

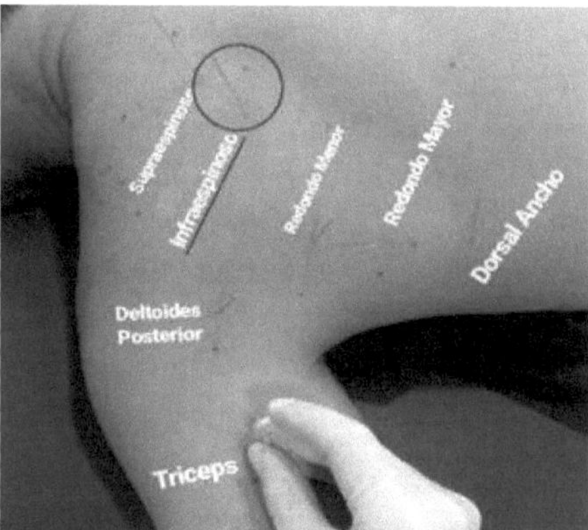

Figure 16. PS needle for infraspinatus in prone position.

- Hazards and Precautions: Risk of pneumothorax and damage to the scapula, especially if there is a congenital malformation (faraminae) that could lead to perforation. It is estimated that between 0.8% and 5.4% of the population has this condition. It is crucial to avoid going too deep with the needle to prevent these risks (89, 90).

4.3.3. Subscapularis.

- Referred pain pattern: The referred pain of subscapularis muscle PGMs is mainly concentrated in the back of the shoulder. This pain may radiate down the back of the arm to the elbow and occasionally cause hyperesthesia or bracelet-like pain around the wrist, especially on the dorsal aspect. Often, a pattern of paresthesia is seen extending throughout the hand, along with pain on the anterior aspect of the shoulder at the level of the tendon, although it is unclear whether this is referred pain or whether there are insertional PGMs.

- Associated symptoms: Patients with subscapularis myofascial pain syndrome (MPS) tend to experience pain both at rest and during movement, often leading to nocturnal discomfort. The shortening of the muscle can cause limitations in mobility, especially in abduction and external rotation. These features make the most likely diagnosis frozen shoulder or adhesive capsulitis.
- PGM activation: Overload situations due to repetitive movements, such as throwing movements in sports, freestyle swimming, shoulder dislocations or fractures, and prolonged periods of immobilization, are some of the possible causes that could activate the PGMs of the subscapularis muscle.
- Related muscles: The teres major, latissimus dorsi and pectoralis major muscles act as agonist muscles, stabilizing the glenohumeral joint, while the infraspinatus and teres minor muscles are antagonists of the subscapularis in its rotator function.
- PS: Given the difficulty of accessing the subscapularis muscle by palpation, dry needling (DS) serves a dual purpose: diagnosis and treatment. There are two approaches to explore and treat the PGMs, the lateral or axillary approach and the medial approach.
    - Axillary approach: This method is considered the safest in several studies. The patient is placed in the supine position with the arm in flexion or in abduction and external rotation. A 0.30 mm x 50 mm needle is used, inserting it laterally towards the anterior aspect of the scapula, ensuring that the needle remains close to the rib cage.

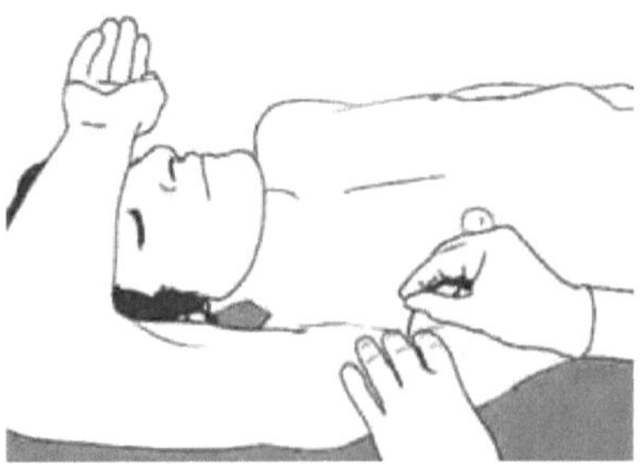

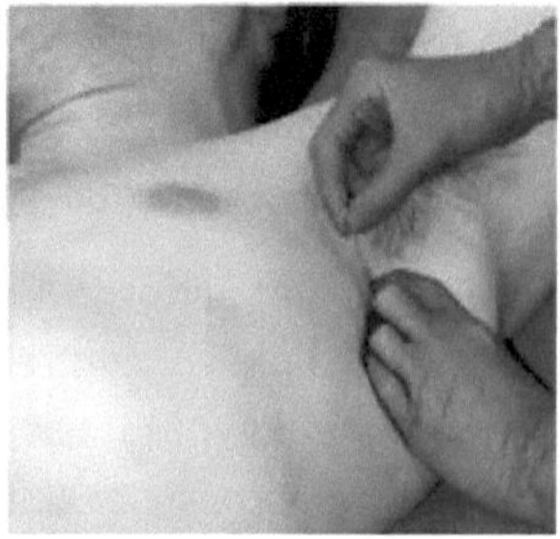

Figure 17. Axillary puncture of the PGMs of the subscapularis muscle (40, 66).

- Medial approach: This approach can be performed in two variants: medial-superior and medial-inferior. In the first, the patient is in homolateral decubitus with the shoulder in flexion and external rotation. In the second, the patient is in prone position, with the shoulder in internal rotation. A needle of at least 0.25 mm x 40 mm is used, curving the needle in the direction of the ventral aspect of the scapula to avoid injury to the lung.

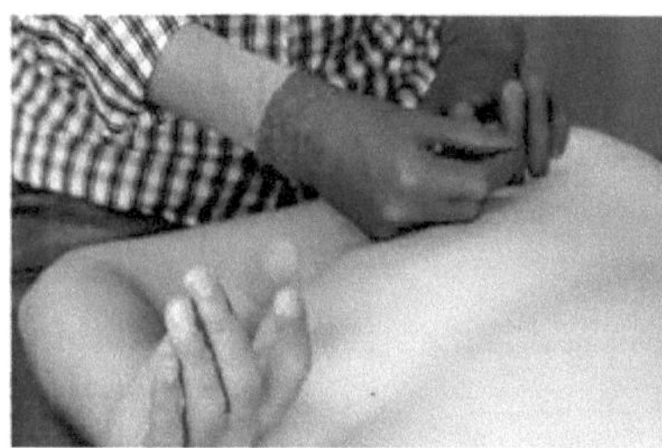
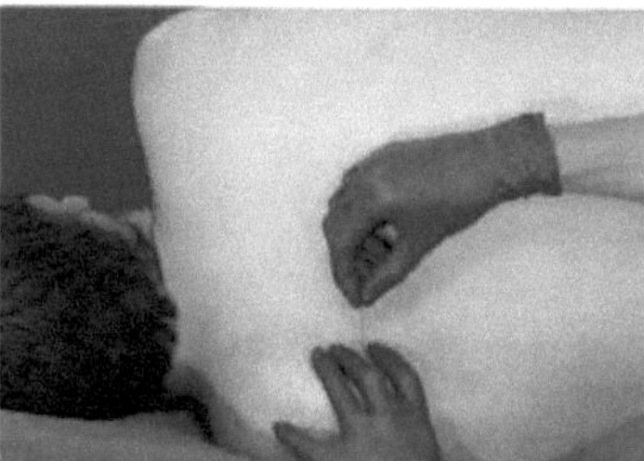

Figure 18. PS by medial approach first figure by medial-superior variant and second figure by medial-inferior variant (66).

- Dangers and Precautions: Invasive treatment of the subscapularis muscle carries several risks, including the possibility of pneumothorax, especially in the medial approach. There is also a risk of damage to adjacent muscles (latissimus dorsi and teres major) or the vasculonervous bundle. It is essential to use ultrasound or electromyographic guidance to minimize these risks. In addition, puncture in patients with coagulation disorders is an absolute contraindication.

4.3.4. Supraspinatus.

- Myofascial trigger points (MTrPs): The supraspinatus muscle can present both central and insertional myofascial trigger points. Insertional trigger points are located at the myotendinous junction or at the tendinoperiosteal insertion. An MTrP can also be found in the body of the tendon, which is also classified as insertional (88, 89, 90).
- Referred pain and symptoms: Central PGMs usually cause deep pain in the shoulder that extends to the medial deltoid region and may radiate to the lateral aspect of the arm and forearm, without reaching

the wrist. Occasionally, the pain may be felt in the epicondyle, which may suggest epicondylitis or lateral epicondylalgia. Insertional PGMs concentrate pain around the "stump" of the shoulder. These points often lead to diagnoses of rotator cuff tendinopathies or subdeltoid bursitis. In addition, patients often present with pain both during physical activity and at rest. The pain is especially noticeable during abduction motion or when the patient holds the arm in that position (88, 89, 90).

- Activation mechanisms: The supraspinatus muscle can be activated and develop PGM in situations such as overloading by heavy loads hanging from the arm, hyperactivity of muscles such as latissimus dorsi or pectoralis major, repetitive overhead movements such as in sports or work activities, direct trauma to the shoulder region (88, 89, 90).
- Treatment by dry needling (88, 89, 90):
  - For central PGMs located in the supraspinous fossa, the patient is placed in contralateral lateral decubitus with the arm close to the body and the shoulder elevated. The physiotherapist introduces a 0.30 mm x 50 mm needle in a craniocaudal direction and slightly forward facing.
  - For insertional PGMs on the tendon, the patient should be in internal rotation, extension and adduction, with the hand and forearm behind the body. A 0.25 mm x 25 mm needle is used.

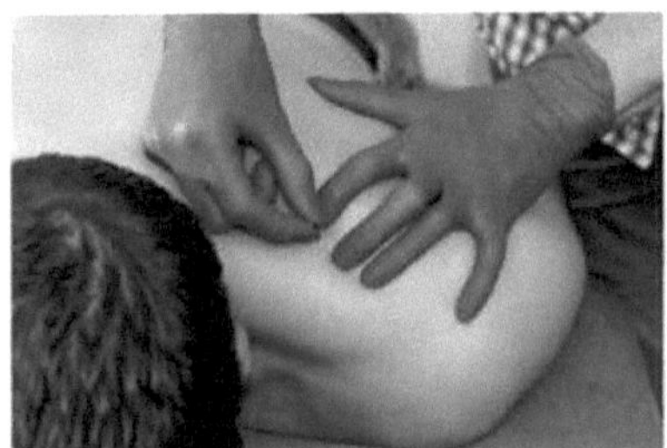
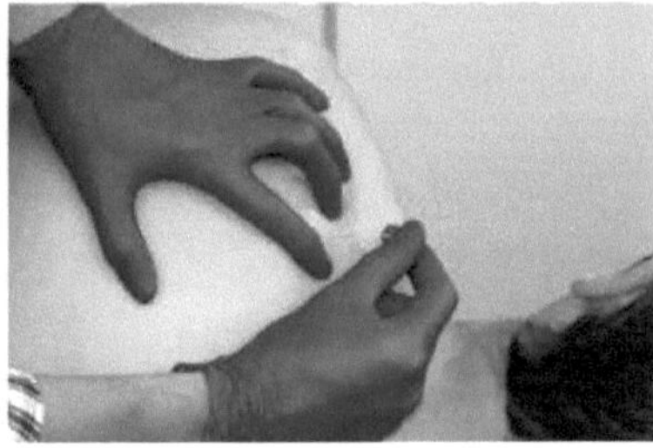

Figure 19. PS in PGM in supraspinatus in prone and lateral decubitus (66).

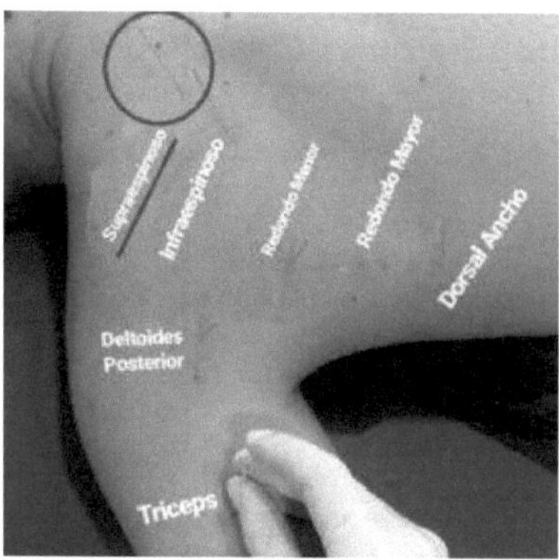

Figure 20. PS for PGM in supraspinatus.

- Important precautions (88, 89, 90):
  - Risk of pneumothorax: Special care in PGMs located in the supraspinous fossa, elevating the scapula to prevent the needle from penetrating the thorax.
  - Rigorous asepsis in the puncture of the insertional PGMs of the tendon due to the proximity to the subacromial bursa or articular cavity.

4.3.5. Deltoid.

- Distribution and location of MTPs: Myofascial trigger points (MTrPs) of the deltoid muscle can be found in the different sections of this muscle, which include the anterior, middle and posterior divisions. These MTrPs are usually located preferentially in the middle part of the anterior and posterior divisions, while in the medial portion, due to the multipenniform configuration of the muscle, they can appear along its entire length (91, 92).
- The pattern of referred pain varies according to the affected section of the muscle (91, 92):
  - Anterior fibers: Pain is localized in the anterior and medial part of the shoulder.
  - Middle fibers: Pain radiates to the lateral aspect of the shoulder, extending slightly to adjacent areas.
  - Posterior fibers: They generate pain in the back of the shoulder, with a slight overflow to the back of the arm and the anterior area of the same. In some cases, this pain pattern may extend into the

upper trapezius and down the back of the arm, almost to the elbow.

- Symptoms: Patients with deltoid MMP usually report pain during movement and rarely at rest. In addition, they may have weakness and inability to perform certain movements, such as shoulder abduction. In some cases, anterior deltoid MMPs may generate a painful locking or "catching" sensation around 15° of abduction, which may be due to simultaneous dysfunction of the supraspinatus muscle. Posterior deltoid involvement may limit movements such as internal rotation and adduction (e.g., when reaching posteriorly). These PGMs may also alter reciprocal inhibition between antagonist muscles, resulting in delayed relaxation of antagonist muscles and compromised control of voluntary movement (91, 92).
- Activation mechanisms: PGMs in the deltoid can be activated by direct trauma, overload in repetitive activities, or in relation to PGMs in adjacent muscles. Deltoid MMPs have been found in 50% of patients with nonspecific shoulder pain. The location of this muscle, which is in the reference area of other MMPs, makes it prone to secondary activation by key MMPs in muscles such as the supraspinatus or trapezius (91, 92).
- PS: Treatment of MMPs in the deltoid by dry needling is relatively simple. The following is a detailed approach according to the affected portion of the muscle (91, 92).
  - Anterior fibers: It is treated with the patient in the supine position. The flat palpation technique can be used, where the needle (0.25 mm x 25 mm) is inserted anteroposteriorly until contacting the humerus. Alternatively, in some patients, the anterior deltoid may be treated with pincer palpation, in which case the needle is inserted mediolaterally.
  - Medial fibers: The ideal position is lateral decubitus on the healthy side, with the arm alongside the body. The needle is directed towards the humerus in a lateromedial direction, using a 0.30 mm x 40 mm needle if necessary.
  - Posterior fibers: This can be approached with the patient in lateral or prone position, with the shoulder in 90° flexion. Another option is to place the patient in lateral decubitus with the arm in internal rotation and abduction, resting the hand on the posterior pelvis,

which facilitates localization of the PGM in the posterior fibers of the muscle.

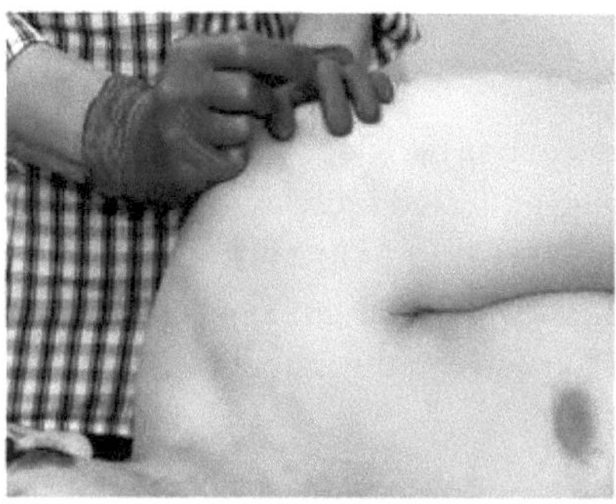

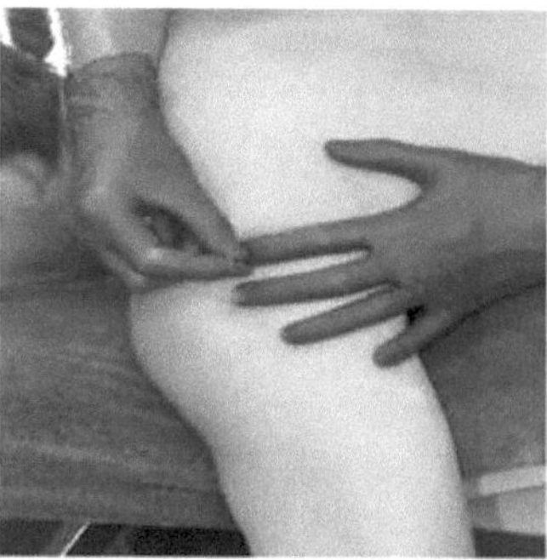

Figure 21. PS of the middle part of the deltoid muscle with the patient in lateral decubitus and PS of the posterior part of the deltoid muscle with the patient in prone decubitus (66).

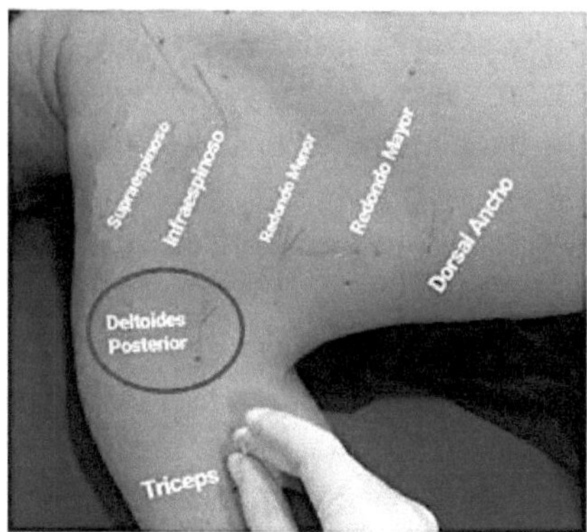

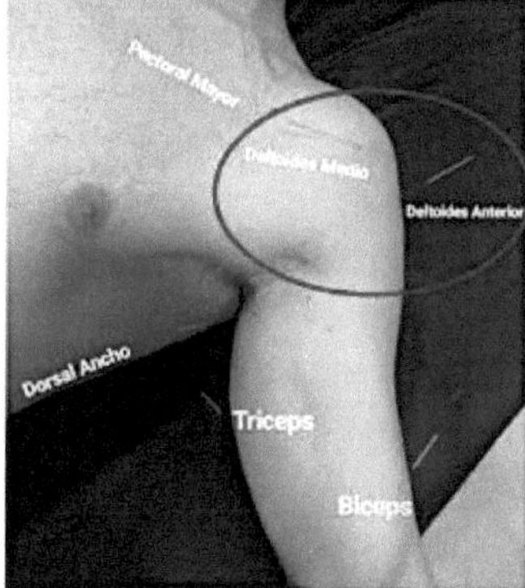

Figure 22. PS of the posterior part of the deltoid muscle with the patient in prone position and PS for middle and anterior deltoid in supine position.

- Precautions and hazards When performing dry needling of the deltoid, there are certain risks to be considered (91, 92):
  - Joint capsule and joint: There is a possibility of the needle passing through the joint capsule if the PGM is close to the joint, so extreme asepsis is recommended.
  - Cephalic vein: During the approach to the anterior fibers, the needle may come into contact with the cephalic vein, so it is

important to direct it away from the location of this vessel and to perform prolonged compression after puncture to avoid hematomas.

4.3.6. Minor round.

- Location of the MTrPs: The teres minor muscle, according to Simons et al. is one of the least frequently affected muscles in the shoulder region. Myofascial trigger points (MTrPs) in this muscle are located between the infraspinatus superiorly and the teres major inferiorly, generally located between its insertions on the scapula and humerus (93, 94, 95).
- Referred pain: pain related to the teres minor teres PGMs is felt in the back of the shoulder at the posterior deltoid insertion area and may extend mildly into the back of the arm. Patients may also experience dysesthesias, such as tingling or numbness in the fourth and fifth fingers (93, 94, 95).
- Symptoms: The main symptoms in patients with active PGMs in the lesser round muscle include (93, 94, 95):
  - Pain: This is more noticeable than limited mobility and increases when the muscle is contracted or stretched. Activities such as reaching behind the body, climbing gestures or movements such as arming the arm to throw tend to exacerbate the pain.
  - Palpable thickening: Patients may feel a thickening in the painful area, which sometimes leads to misdiagnosis as subdeltoid bursitis.
  - Atrophy and instability: The teres minor muscle may atrophy in some cases of shoulder pain, affecting up to 3% of patients. This lesion is related to quadrangular space syndrome and axillary nerve entrapment, which may be due to anatomical variations of the muscle or nerve trunk.
- Trigger mechanisms: Movements that cause contractions in shortening or stretching of the teres minor muscle, such as gestures of external rotation and horizontal adduction of the shoulder, are the main triggers of pain. This muscle works in conjunction with the infraspinatus, posterior deltoid and the rest of the rotator cuff muscles, mainly in external rotation and stabilization of the

glenohumeral joint. Antagonist muscles of the teres minor include the subscapularis, pectoralis major, and anterior deltoid (93, 94, 95).

- PS: Dry needling treatment for the PGMs of the teres minor follows a procedure similar to that described for the infraspinatus muscle. The use of a 0.30 mm x 40 mm needle is recommended and is performed with care to follow the correct direction of the needle toward the scapula (93, 94, 95).

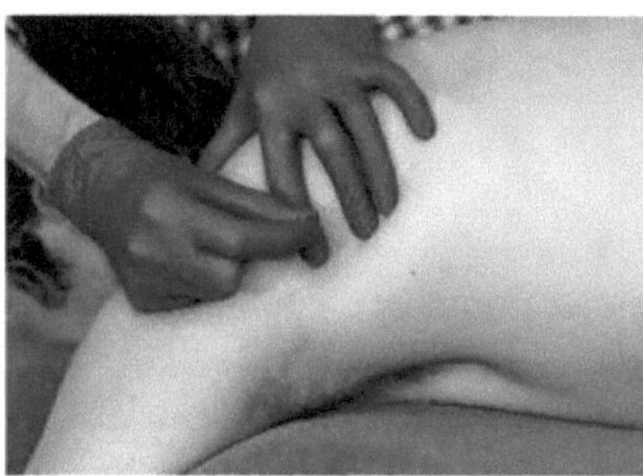

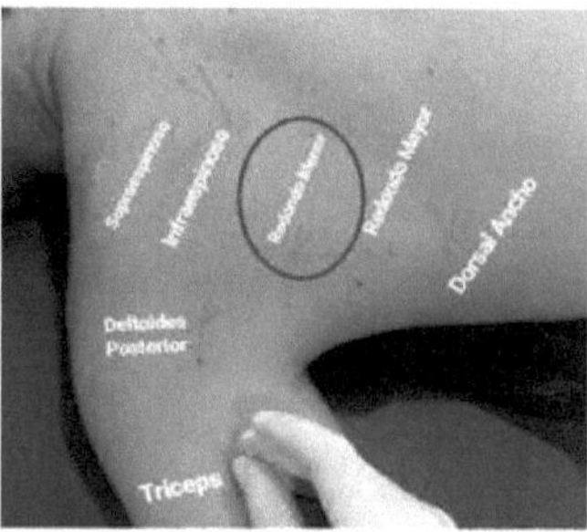

Figure 23. PS of the teres minor muscle with the patient in prone position (66).

- Dangers and precautions: When performing dry needling in the teres minor, the risk of pneumothorax must be taken into account, especially in patients with considerable muscle volume, where palpation may be less precise. To avoid this, it is important to direct the needle parallel to the plane of the scapula, making sure that it does not cross into the thorax (93, 94, 95).

4.3.7. Larger round.

- Location and activation of MTPs: Active myofascial trigger points (MTrPs) of the teres major muscle are important causes of pain in the shoulder region. Pain presents in the posterolateral aspect of the shoulder and may radiate along the posterior arm and forearm. Although isolated structural lesions in this muscle are rare, they are usually the result of trauma. Patients may experience pain in the back of the shoulder, accompanied by limitation of mobility, especially in abduction, external rotation and flexion movements. In addition, there may be weakness in internal rotation and extension of the shoulder (94, 95).

- Symptoms and activities that activate PGMs: PGMs of the teres major tend to manifest when the patient performs activities that require a shortening contraction of the muscle, such as climbing or pulling a rope. These activities that combine overhead arm elevation or movements in which the muscle is shortened can trigger pain. Causes that can lead to the onset of PGMs in the teres major round include: Repetitive movements, trauma to the shoulder region, periods of immobilization, degenerative processes. PGMs of the teres major may also be observed in patients with adhesive capsulitis or radiculopathies. In addition, this muscle plays a role in the quadrangular space syndrome of the shoulder, first described in 1983 by Cahill and Palmer, where pain presents with paresthesias in the posterior part of the shoulder due to possible compression of the neurovascular bundle in the quadrangular space (94, 95).
- Referred pain pattern: The referred pain pattern in teres major PGMs includes localized pain in the posterior aspect of the shoulder, which may extend to the posterior arm and forearm. This pattern is common with movements requiring abduction and external rotation of the shoulder (94, 95).
- Related muscles: The teres major works together with the latissimus dorsi and triceps brachii (long portion), being agonists in the extension and internal rotation movements of the shoulder (94, 95).
- PS in the teres major: Invasive treatment of the PGMs of the teres major is performed using the clamp puncture technique. The anatomical position of the muscle facilitates this approach. Although it is possible to perform the technique with the patient in the supine position, the recommended positions are lateral decubitus or prone decubitus (94, 95).
    - Lateral decubitus: The patient is placed in lateral decubitus on the healthy side, holding the affected arm in a 90° flexion and internal rotation position. The scapula is moved forward to facilitate access to the muscle, allowing the physical therapist to grasp the muscle in a clamp. A 0.30 mm x 50 mm needle is used, which is inserted in the direction of the finger opposite the grip and the taut band.
    - Prone: The patient drops the affected arm outside of the table, allowing gravity to pull the scapula down, facilitating access to the muscle. Alternatively, the patient's forearm may rest on a stool or armrest for comfort.

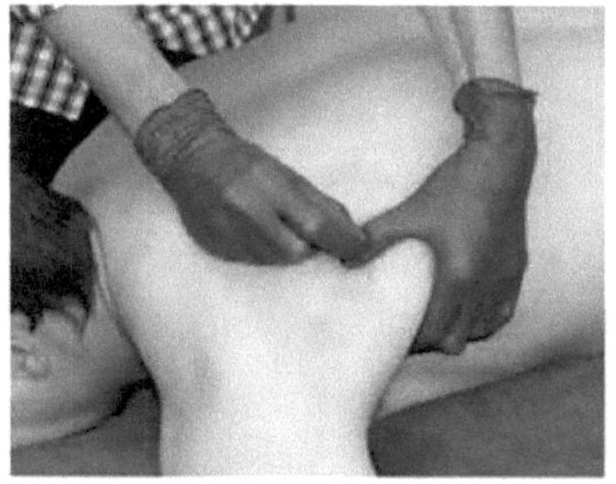

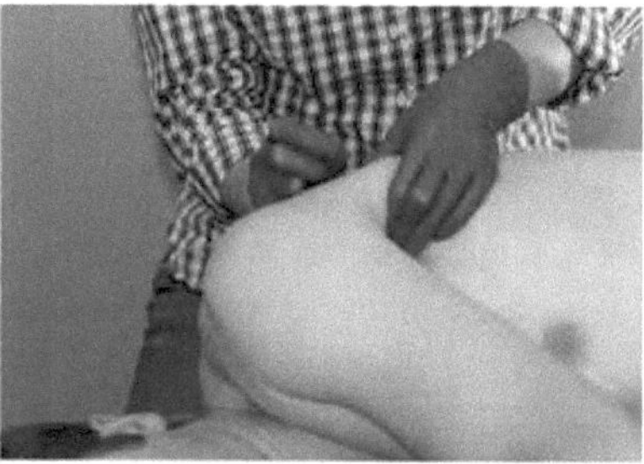

Figure 24. PS for teres major in prone and lateral decubitus (66).

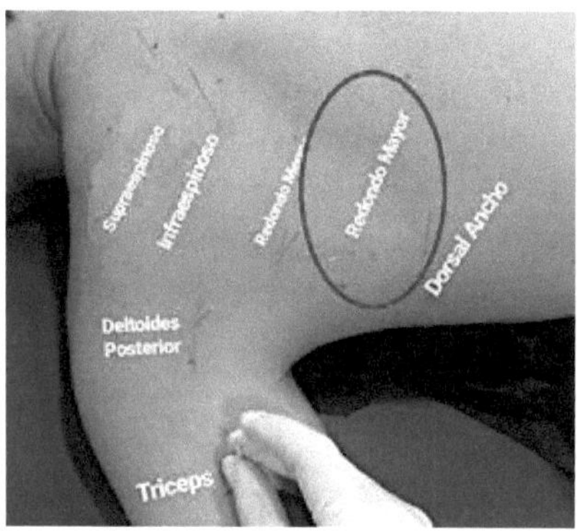

Figure 25. PS for teres major in prone position.

- Dangers and precautions: Due to its anatomic location, dry needling in the greater round carries risks of complications such as pneumothorax. However, this risk is minimized by using the clamp puncture technique. In addition, it is important to be careful with the neurovascular bundle, as the PGMs located on the lateral side of the muscle may be close to the axillary nerve and circumflex artery, both of which cross the posterior quadrangular space of the shoulder (94, 95).

4.3.8. Broad dorsal.

- Location and activation of MTPs: The latissimus dorsi muscle is usually affected by myofascial trigger points (MTPs) in its most cranial fibers, near the lateral border of the scapula and the posterior axillary crease. It is less common to find MTPs in its more vertical and anterior fibers. The latissimus dorsi PGMs can produce pain centered in the middorsal region, which is often ignored as a cause of back pain (96, 97, 98).

- Referred pain patterns (96, 97, 98):
  - Superior (horizontal) fibers: Pain projects to the back of the scapula, upper arm, forearm, and fourth and fifth fingers. In these cases, patients tend to experience paresthesias and numbness rather than pain.
  - Inferior (vertical) fibers: Pain is located on the anterior aspect of the shoulder and on the inferolateral aspect of the trunk, just above the iliac crest.
  - Intermediate (oblique) fibers: May cause pain in the posterior axillary crease, outside the scapula.
- Associated symptoms and activities that activate PGMs: Patients with latissimus dorsi PGMs often present with back pain in the dorsal region, with stinging or burning sensations that make it difficult to find a comfortable position. Discomfort is often increased when stretching the muscle, such as when pushing an object forward or performing shortened contractions, such as in pull-ups, climbing or personal hygiene (96, 97, 98).
- Causes of MGPs: Causes that may cause MGPs in latissimus dorsi include muscle overload from activities such as climbing, rowing, tennis or gymnastics, MGPs in the serratus posterior superior or subscapularis, wearing tight clothing such as a very tight bra, shoulder surgeries, radiculopathies of the roots that innervate the muscle (96, 97, 98).
- Related muscles (96, 97, 98):
  - Agonists: The latissimus dorsi works together with the teres major, the long head of the triceps (in shoulder abduction) and the abdominal fibers of the pectoralis major in the extension and internal rotation of the shoulder.
  - Antagonists: the upper trapezius in relation to the shoulder, the triceps brachii (long head) when the arm is alongside the body, and the scalenes in relation to the thorax.
- PS in the latissimus dorsi muscle: The dry needling technique in latissimus dorsi varies according to the affected area, either the most proximal (upper fibers) or the most distal (lower fibers) (96, 97, 98).

- Superior fibers (horizontal): It is treated through a clamp puncture, similar to the technique used for the teres major. Patient position in lateral or prone decubitus. Another option is to perform the puncture with the patient in supine decubitus, with the shoulder in abduction of about 90° and external rotation (96, 97, 98).
- Vertical fibers: If the MGP can be palpated and clamped, the puncture is simple and can be performed with the patient in lateral decubitus. It is important to ensure that the needle is kept inside the clamp to avoid the risk of pneumothorax. If the PGM cannot be clamped, the puncture should be performed by placing the taut band over a rib. The needle should be introduced tangentially to the thorax to avoid puncturing it (96, 97, 98).

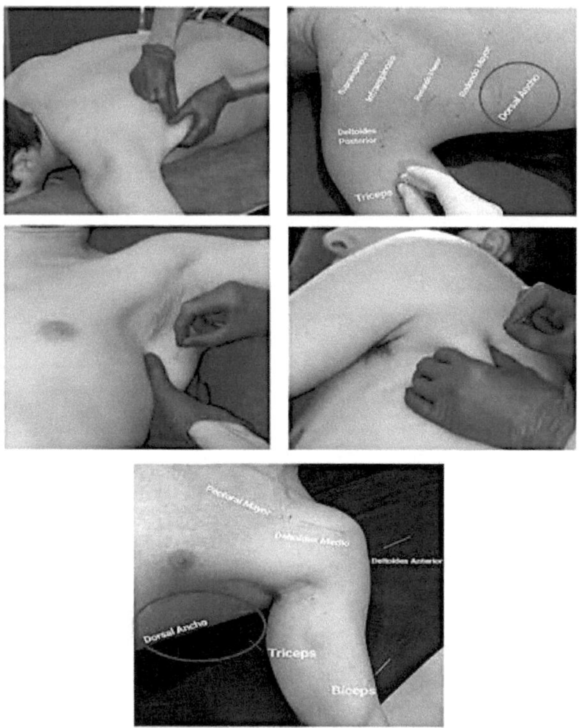

Figure 26. PS for PGM in latissimus dorsi in prone, supine and lateral decubitus (66).

- Dangers and precautions: It is essential to follow the necessary precautions to avoid complications such as pneumothorax. In punctures where the PGM cannot be palpated in forceps, the puncture should be performed with extreme care, ensuring that the needle follows the curvature of the thorax and remains tangential to the bony structure. In addition, short needle lengths are recommended to minimize the risk of perforation (96, 97, 98).

4.3.9. Major and minor rhomboids.

- Location and activation of MTrPs: Myofascial trigger points (MTrPs) in the greater and lesser rhomboid muscles are mainly located medially, between their vertebral and scapular insertions. These MTrPs can trigger insertional trigger points, which increase hypersensitivity at the medial border of the scapula (99, 100).
- Referred pain patterns: PGM-referred pain in the rhomboids is typically located in the interscapular region of the affected side, similar to the pattern in muscles such as the levator scapulae and scalenes. This pain often extends to the supraspinous fossa and may be confused with dorsal nerve syndrome of the scapula due to the proximity of motor innervation (99, 100).
- Associated symptoms (99, 100):
    - The patient may experience alterations in the sensitivity of the skin covering the affected area.
    - Crackling and crackling are common in the region.
    - Pain may increase when the patient is in homolateral decubitus (leaning on the affected side).
    - Clinically, the pain is often superficial at rest, without clear mechanical characteristics.
- Causes of PGM activation: PGMs in the rhomboids are not very common in isolation and are usually related to postural factors. The most frequent causes include rounded shoulder postures, maintained for long periods, generate considerable muscle overload. This is intensified when the shoulder is held in prolonged abduction or flexion to 90 degrees. In turn, conditions such as scoliosis or having undergone thoracic surgery can aggravate this situation. In addition, weakness of the serratus anterior muscle contributes to instability of the region, while shortening of muscles such as the pectoralis major further limits shoulder mobility and functionality (99, 100).

- Related muscles (99, 100):
  - Synergistic: The levator scapulae and upper trapezius collaborate in scapular elevation. The levator scapulae and latissimus dorsi assist in scapular rotation, while the medial trapezius participates in adduction of the scapula together with the rhomboids.
  - Antagonists: The serratus anterior and pectoralis major act in opposition to the rhomboids.
- Treatment with PS: Treatment with PS in the rhomboids depends on the location of the PGMs. There are three recommended positions for the patient (99, 100):
  - PGM near the vertebral border of the scapula: In these cases, it is important to detach the scapula from the ribs in order to introduce the needle tangentially to the thorax, thus avoiding the risk of pneumothorax. The lateral decubitus position on the affected side can be used to treat the PGMs of the lesser rhomboid or the prone position, with the patient's hand behind the waist, to treat the greater rhomboid.
  - PGM in the central part of the rhomboids: The best option is to place the patient in prone position, and the physical therapist should palpate the tense band of the muscle from below, directing the needle as tangential as possible to the ribs. In all cases, it is recommended to use a 0.25 mm x 25 mm needle.

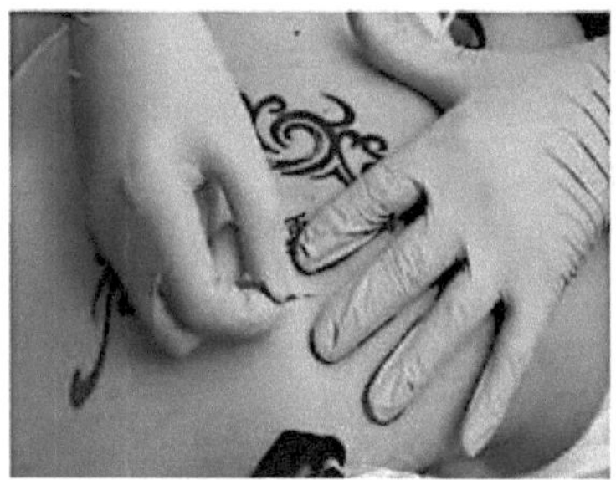

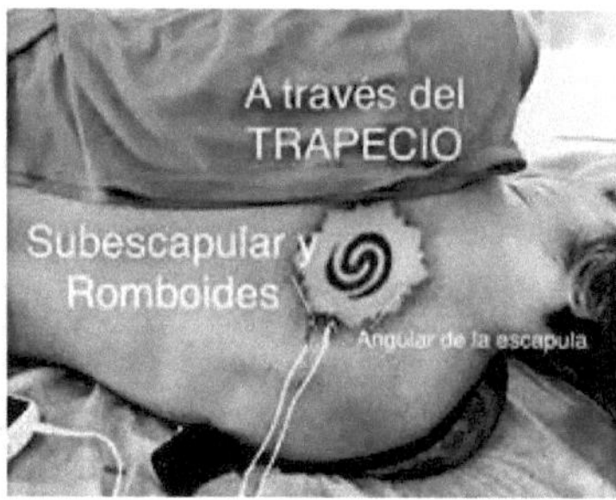

Figure 27. PS for PGM in rhomboid with patient in prone position (66).

- Dangers and precautions: The risk of pneumothorax can be avoided by following the indications described for patient positioning and needle direction during puncture. Correct technique, especially when detaching the scapula from the ribs and directing the needle tangentially, is essential to prevent complications (99, 100).

4.4. Muscle of the arm, forearm and hand.

4.4.1. Biceps brachii.

- Location of MTrPs: Myofascial trigger points (MTrPs) in the biceps brachii muscle are usually located medially, and their referred pain pattern tends to project proximally, which is unusual compared to other muscles (101, 102).
- Referred pain patterns: The most frequent referred pain from biceps MGPs occurs in the anterior deltoid region and ulnar fossa. Occasionally, it may project to the suprascapular region or upper trapezius. This pattern of superficial anterior deltoid pain can lead to diagnostic confusion, such as possible tenosynovitis of the long head of the biceps. Palpation of the tendon may also be painful due to tension in the area, complicating the differential diagnosis. Additionally, the presence of PGM in the short head of the biceps can generate pain in the coracoid process, although it is not clear whether this is referred pain or an enthesopathy (insertional PGM) (101, 102).
- Associated symptoms (101, 102):
  - Pain in the anterior deltoid region and ulnar fossa.
  - Pain may worsen when performing activities that involve shoulder flexion above 90º.
  - Increased tension due to PGMs can lead to enthesopathies in the biceps tendon, causing pain in shoulder abductions between 15º and 20º.
  - In less frequent cases, pain in the coracoid process related to the short head of the biceps may occur.
- PGMs in the biceps can be activated in several ways (101, 102):
  - Direct mechanisms:
    - Excessive flexion of the elbow in supination (such as when carrying loads with the elbow flexed).
    - Repetitive supination activities (use of screwdrivers).
    - Eccentric overload, such as when holding a railing with the elbow straight to avoid a fall.
  - Indirect mechanisms:
    - Alterations in the glenohumeral joint, such as anterior instability.
    - Prolonged immobilization of the elbow.

- PGMs in muscles such as the scalenes or infraspinatus, which are often key to the activation and resolution of biceps PGMs.
- Certain sports activities, such as bowling or tennis, also favor the appearance of PGMs in this muscle.

- Related muscles: scalenes, infraspinatus, coracobrachialis, subclavian and brachialis (101, 102).
- Treatment with PS: Dry needling treatment of the biceps brachii is performed with the patient in the supine position, with the shoulder in 45º abduction and the elbow in 45º flexion. The physiotherapist is positioned lateral to the patient's arm (101, 102).
  - Long head of the biceps: The taut bands are palpated and the needle is introduced anteroposteriorly, also crossing the brachialis muscle to treat possible PGMs in this muscle. A 0.25 mm x 40 mm needle is recommended.

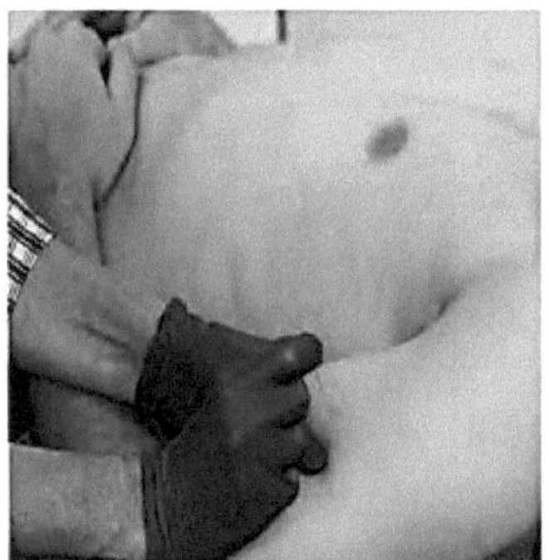

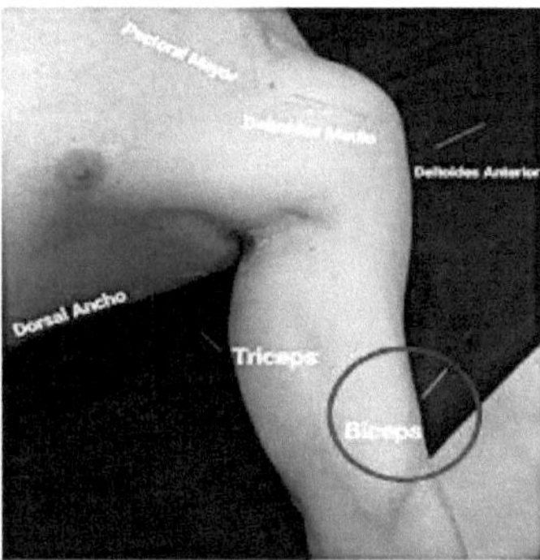

Figure 28. PS for PGM in long head of the biceps brachii (66).

  - Short head of the biceps: A clamp palpation is used to isolate the short head and the needle is introduced in a lateral-medial or medial-lateral fashion.

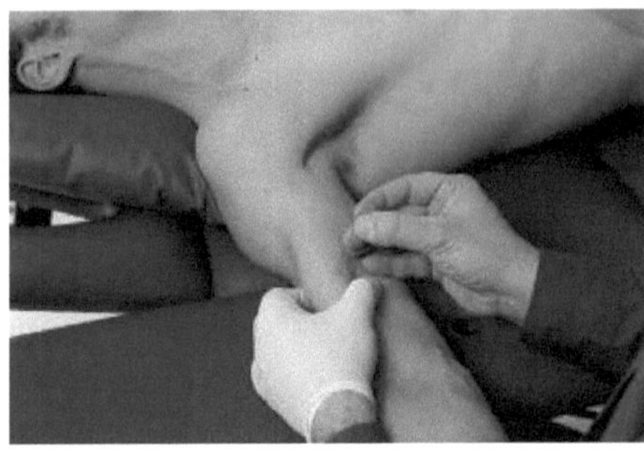

Figure 29. PS for PGM in short head of the biceps brachii (66).

- Dangers and precautions: When performing dry needling of the biceps, it is important to be aware of the proximity of the radial and median nerves, which run along the lateral and medial borders, respectively, of the biceps and brachialis. Necessary precautions should be followed to avoid accidental nerve puncture (101, 102).

4.4.2. Coracobrachial.

- Location of MTPs: Myofascial trigger points (MTPs) in the coracobrachialis muscle are located in its central part and their referred pain pattern is mainly projected on the anterior aspect of the shoulder (over the anterior deltoid) and in the posterolateral region of the arm, forearm and hand, sometimes extending to the dorsum of the middle finger, without directly affecting the elbow and wrist joints (103, 104).
- Referred pain patterns: Pain referred to the anterior aspect of the shoulder is usually reproduced when the patient performs the gesture of actively bringing the hand to the back. This feature may lead to diagnostic confusion as it may mimic other shoulder disorders (103, 104).
- Musculocutaneous nerve relationship: The musculocutaneous nerve passes through the coracobrachialis muscle before innervating the biceps and brachialis. The presence of MGP in the coracobrachialis could result in compression or entrapment of the nerve, which could lead to atrophy of the biceps and brachialis, loss of strength in elbow flexion and even a decrease or abolition of the bicipital reflex. This situation has been documented in cases of coracobrachial hypertrophy (103, 104).

- Associated symptoms (103, 104):
  - Pain in the anterior aspect of the shoulder.
  - Pain in the posterolateral aspect of the arm, forearm and hand, with the possibility of extension to the dorsum of the middle finger.
  - Entrapment of the musculocutaneous nerve, which can lead to atrophy and loss of strength in the muscles innervated by this nerve.
- Mechanisms of PGM activation: PGMs in the coracobrachialis are usually activated secondarily due to the presence of PGMs in other functionally related muscles, such as (103, 104):
  - Agonists: Pectoralis major, anterior deltoid, short head of biceps brachii.
  - Antagonists: posterior deltoid, long head of triceps, latissimus dorsi, teres major.
  - Key proximal muscles: Scalenes, which may be critical for the activation and resolution of PGMs in the coracobrachialis.
- Related muscles (103, 104):
  - Agonists and related muscles: anterior deltoid, short head of biceps, pectoralis major.
  - Antagonists and related muscles: latissimus dorsi, teres major, long head of triceps, posterior deltoid.
- Treatment with PS: Dry needling treatment of the coracobrachialis is a favorable therapeutic option due to the difficulty of accessing the muscle for conservative manual techniques. Great care must be taken due to the proximity of the neurovascular bundle and the presence of the musculocutaneous nerve (103, 104).
  - Patient position: The patient should be positioned in supine decubitus, with the shoulder in abduction close to 90º and in internal rotation, while the forearm rests on the stretcher with the elbow in 90º flexion.
  - Palpation and localization: To palpate the PGMs of the coracobrachialis, the short head of the biceps, which is caudal to the anterior axillary crease and medial to the anterior deltoid, is taken as a reference. The coracobrachialis is immediately dorsal to the short head of the biceps. It is differentiated by contraction of the coracobrachialis by requesting

shoulder adduction, in which simultaneous contraction of the biceps and coracobrachialis is perceived. If no contraction is seen in this maneuver, the neurovascular bundle is most likely involved.

- Puncture: Once the PGM is located, the taut band is stabilized by flat palpation against the humerus. A 0.25 mm x 40 mm needle is introduced and directed parallel to the plane of the stretcher, seeking contact with the humerus.

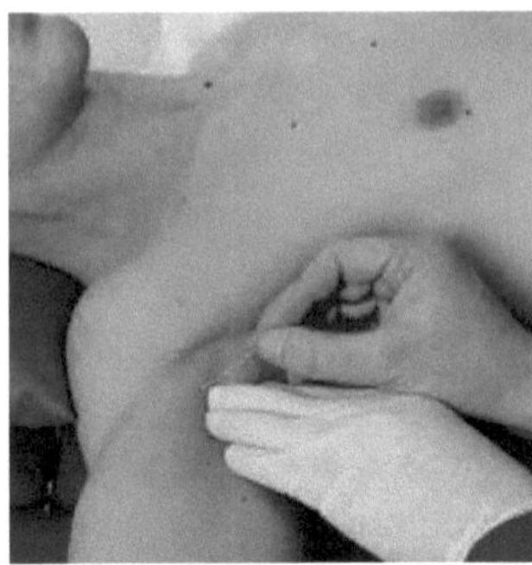

Figure 30. PS in PGM for coracobrachial (66).

- Hazards and Precautions: Because the musculocutaneous nerve runs through the muscular belly of the coracobrachialis, the usual guidelines should be followed to avoid injuring the nerve. The neurovascular bundle, which includes the median and ulnar nerve and the brachial artery, is dorsal to the coracobrachial, so medial orientation of the needle should be avoided. To minimize risks we should request shoulder adduction to confirm coracobrachial contracture and ensure that the needle is directed anteroposteriorly and not medially toward the neurovascular bundle (103, 104).

4.4.3. Triceps.

Myofascial trigger points (MTrPs) in the triceps brachii can be divided into different zones depending on the muscle head where they are located. Each zone projects a specific referred pain pattern (105, 106):

- PGM in the long head of the triceps:
    - Located mainly in the proximal half of the muscle.
    - Referred pain from the PGM area to the dorsal aspect of the shoulder and may reach the upper trapezius.

- Pain may also extend to the lateral epicondyle region and posterior forearm.

- PGM at the lateral head of the triceps:
  - Commonly located in the central part of the lateral head.
  - The pain is usually localized in the area of the PGMs, mainly in the posterolateral aspect of the arm.
  - In some cases, the pain may radiate to the dorsum of the forearm and affect the fourth and fifth fingers.
  - There may be radial nerve entrapment, causing sensory disturbances in the posterior and lateral part of the forearm.
- PGM at the medial head of the triceps:
  - Lateral fibers: project pain to the lateral epicondyle and lateral forearm.
  - Central and distal fibers: cause pain in the olecranon (according to Simons) or more frequently in the medial epicondyle, depending on the authors.
  - Medial fibers: cause pain in the epitrochlea and may radiate towards the inner part of the forearm, sometimes reaching the palmar part of the fourth and fifth fingers.
- Common symptoms (105, 106):
  - Pain in the lateral epicondyle and ulnar region of the forearm and hand.
  - Pain in the dorsal aspect of the shoulder and upper trapezius.
  - Sensation of weakness in elbow extension.
  - Possibility of nerve entrapment (radial or ulnar), with sensory alterations.
- Activation mechanisms (105, 106):
  - Movements that involve repetitive elbow extension, such as push-ups, excessive weight training, tennis, golf, boxing or acrobatic activities.
  - Activities with arms held in front of the body without elbow support (physiotherapy, driving, office work).
  - Indirect activation by key PGMs in other related muscles such as the scalenes, latissimus dorsi, or rounds.
- Dry needling: Dry needling is a recommended technique for the treatment of triceps PGMs. Depending on the muscle head where the PGMs are located, a specific technique is used to avoid nearby nerve

structures, such as the radial and ulnar nerves, and a correct differential palpation should always be performed before inserting the needle (105, 106).

- Long head: Clamp puncture, with 0.30 mm x 50 mm needle.
- Lateral and medial head: 0.25 mm x 40 mm or 0.30 mm x 40 mm needles are used, depending on the location, avoiding nerve structures such as the radial or ulnar nerve.

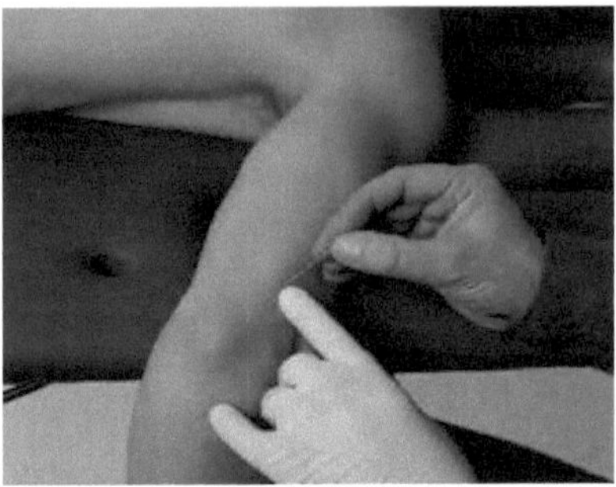

Figure 31. PS in PGM of the lower portion of the triceps in supine decubitus (40, 66).

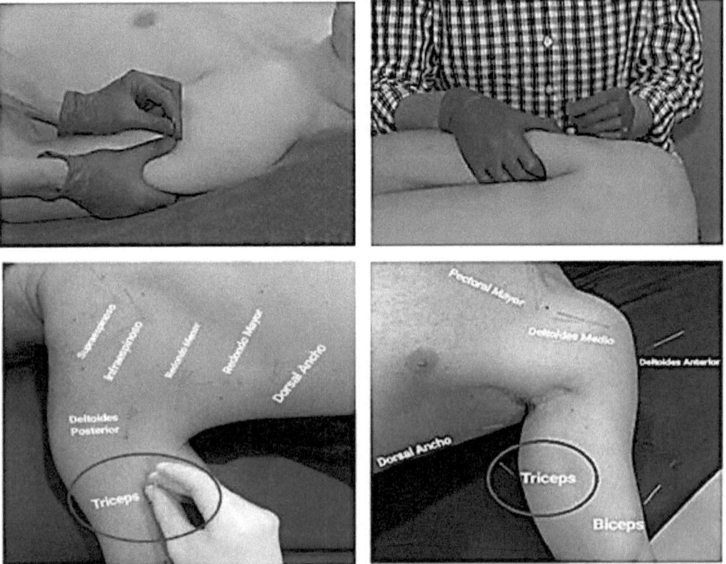

Figure 32. PS in PGM of the triceps brachii in prone, supine and lateral decubitus (66).

- Dangers and precautions: In certain areas of the triceps there is a possibility of touching the radial and ulnar nerves with the needle (105, 106).

4.4.4. Anconeo.

- MGPs of the anconeus: MGPs in the anconeus muscle often report pain and hypersensitivity at the posterior aspect of the lateral epicondyle. This pain pattern may contribute to cases of lateral epicondylalgia in which the pain is located posteriorly, rather than anteriorly, which is the most common location (107, 108).
- Symptoms (107, 108):
  - Localized pain in the posterior part of the lateral epicondyle.
  - Sensitivity to touch in that area.
  - Close functional relationship with the triceps brachii and extensor digitorum, which may amplify pain in activities involving repetitive elbow and finger movements.
- Activation mechanisms (107, 108):
  - Repetitive movements of the index finger: This can cause the PGMs in the ankles to be activated in people who work long hours with keyboard and mouse.
  - Trauma: The anconeus acts as an elbow varus stabilizer, so trauma involving varus forces can induce PGMs in this muscle.
- Muscle relations (107, 108):
  - Muscle tension in antagonists such as the biceps brachii, brachialis, and pronator teres, which stabilizes elbow valgus, can trigger the onset of PGMs in the anconeus.
  - The presence of PGMs in the triceps brachii or in the extensor digitorum (especially the fascicle corresponding to the index finger) may also be a cause of PGMs in the anconeus.
- Related muscles (107, 108): triceps brachii, extensor digitorum, biceps brachii, brachialis and pronator teres.
- Anconeus PS: The following technique is used to treat the PGMs of the anconeus muscle with dry needling (107, 108).
  - Patient position: Supine decubitus with the shoulder slightly abducted and the elbow in 45° flexion, with the forearm in pronation supported on a pillow. It can also be placed in

contralateral decubitus with the elbow flexed and supported on the trunk.

- PGM Location: The PGMs are located slightly caudal to the midpoint between the epicondyle and the olecranon. The taut band is stabilized with flat palpation against the ulna.
- Needle insertion: A 0.25 mm x 25 mm needle is used, and it is inserted in the direction of the lateral border of the ulna.

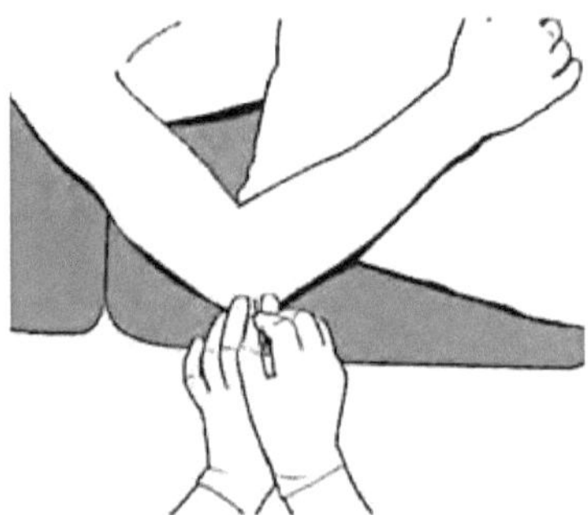
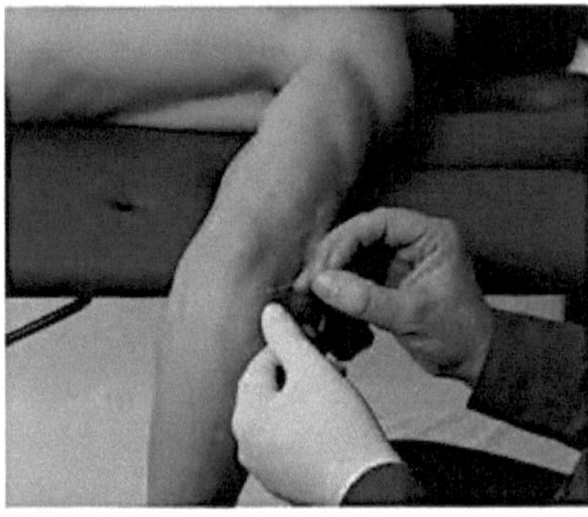

Figure 33. PS in the PGM of the anconeus in supine and prone decubitus (40, 66).

- Hazards and precautions (107, 108):
  - Risk: There is a risk when puncturing this muscle of touching the posterior cutaneous nerve of the forearm, which is a branch of the radial nerve and sometimes runs over the anconeus.
  - Caution: It is important to be careful during needle insertion, especially in the first few millimeters of advancement to avoid contact with the nerve.
- Recommendations: Make sure to identify the nerve by palpation and avoid puncture and maintain a controlled and gradual insertion, observing the patient's reaction.

4.4.5. Brachioradialis.

- Brachioradialis PGMs: Brachioradialis PGMs refer pain and hypersensitivity to the lateral epicondyle and project pain to the base of the thumb and the first interdigital space. This muscle is frequently related to cases of lateral epicondylalgia and its contribution to pain can be significant in activities that require repetitive elbow flexion (109, 110).

- Symptoms: pain and hypersensitivity in the lateral epicondyle, projection of pain towards the base of the thumb and the first interdigital space, tension and tenderness in the proximal forearm (109, 110).
- Activation mechanisms (109, 110):
  - Elbow flexion overload: Activities involving repeated movements or excessive loads in elbow flexion can activate the brachioradialis PGMs.
  - Fractures of the distal third of the radius: In this type of fracture, the brachioradialis may contribute to the displacement of the bony fragment and, in turn, develop PGM.
  - Relationship with other muscles: The brachioradialis often shares PGMs with the supinator, extensor carpi radialis longus and extensor carpi radialis brevis muscles, contributing to the picture of lateral epicondylalgia.
  - Referred pain from proximal muscles: PGMs in muscles such as the infraspinatus, supraspinatus or scalenes can generate secondary PGMs in the brachioradialis.
- Related muscles: Supinator, extensor carpi radialis longus, extensor carpi radialis brevis (109, 110).
- Brachioradialis PS: To perform dry needling in the brachioradialis, the following procedure is followed (109, 110).
  - Muscle localization: The brachioradialis muscle belly can be highlighted by requesting elbow flexion against resistance with the forearm in neutral pronation. It is an easy muscle to palpate, either in pincer or flat, compressing against the radius.
  - Patient position: The patient should be supine with the shoulder slightly abducted and the elbow flexed at about 45°.
  - Needle sizes: For clamp puncture, a 0.25 mm x 25 mm needle is used. For flat puncture, a 0.25 mm x 40 mm needle is recommended. In this case, the radius is used as a reference, and contact with the bone will indicate that both the brachioradialis and extensor carpi radialis longus have been crossed.
  - Technique:
    - Clamp puncture: The PGM is located in the clamp and the needle is directed from one side of the muscle towards the fingers of the opposite side.

- Flat puncture: Flat palpation is recommended to compress the muscle against the radius and guide the puncture to the bone.

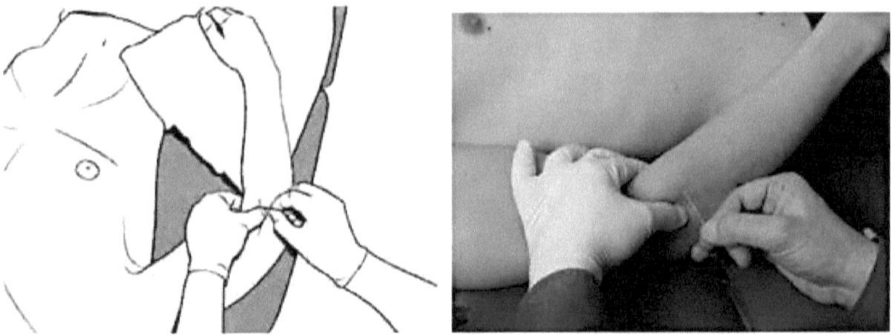

Figure 34. PS in PGM for brachioradialis (40, 66).

- Dangers and precautions: The superficial branch of the radial nerve runs along the posteromedial aspect of the muscle, but the needle is unlikely to contact it if the clamp approach is used. Even so, the usual measures should be followed to avoid complications, especially during the first few millimeters of needle insertion (109, 110).

4.4.6. Radial extensor carpi radialis longus.

- MTPs in the extensor carpi radialis longus: Location and access: The MTPs of this muscle can be palpated directly in clamp or, more deeply, behind the brachioradialis. Pincer palpation is ideal for identifying the muscle and differentiating it from the brachioradialis, as local twitch responses (REL) are obtained on sudden pincer palpation (111, 112).
- Referred pain pattern: The most common pain pattern involves the lateral epicondyle and the dorsum of the hand, specifically in the area of the anatomical clog. The patient with PGM in this muscle frequently experiences pain during hand grip, which is characteristic of lateral epicondylalgia. This pain may increase when performing manual activities such as holding heavy objects or using tools, even in simple movements such as opening a door or picking up a glass (111, 112).
- Symptoms (111, 112):
  - Pain and weakness on wrist extension and grip.
  - Stiffness and difficulty flexing the wrist.
  - Pain when grasping objects or making grasping movements with the hand.
  - Perceptible weakness in the hand and forearm.

- Pain at rest in severe cases.

- Activation mechanisms (111, 112):
  - Repetitive manual activities: Actions involving constant or repeated manual force, such as factory work, cleaning or prolonged keyboard use, can activate PGMs. It is also common in activities involving powerful grips, such as the use of rackets, screwdrivers or butcher knives.
  - Muscle overload: Both acute and chronic muscle overload can generate PGM in the extensor carpi radialis longus.
  - Indirect mechanisms: Cervical conditions (herniated disc, cervical joint dysfunctions) and PGMs in neck and shoulder muscles (especially scalenes, infraspinatus and supraspinatus) can also activate these trigger points.
- Related muscles: extensor carpi radialis brevis, brachioradialis, extensor digitorum, triceps brachii, supinator, scalenes, infraspinatus, supraspinatus (111, 112).
- PS of the extensor carpi radialis longus muscle (111, 112).
  - Patient position: The patient should be supine, with the elbow slightly flexed and the forearm in pronation.
  - Palpation of the muscle: The PGM is palpated in forceps, and is generally located about 4 cm caudal to the lateral epicondyle. The puncture is performed by directing the needle from one side of the muscle towards the opposite fingers, in an anteroposterior direction.
  - Needle size: It is recommended to use a 0.25 mm x 40 mm needle for both clamp puncture (recommended method) and flat palpation.
  - Technique:
    - Clamp puncture: This is the most precise and recommended technique. The muscle is clamped and the needle is introduced towards the fingers on the opposite side.
    - Flat puncture: This is an alternative option, although less precise.

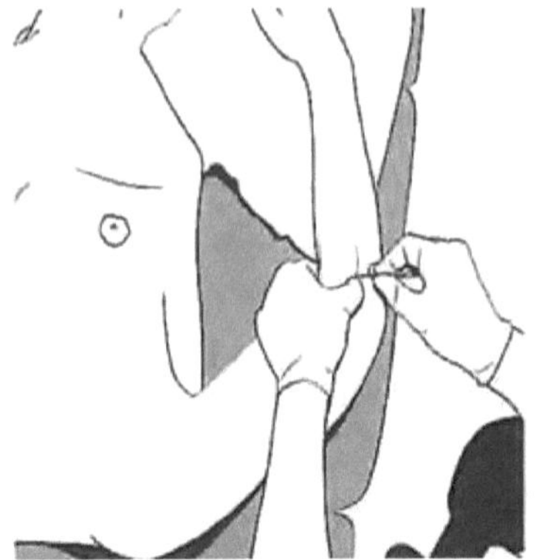

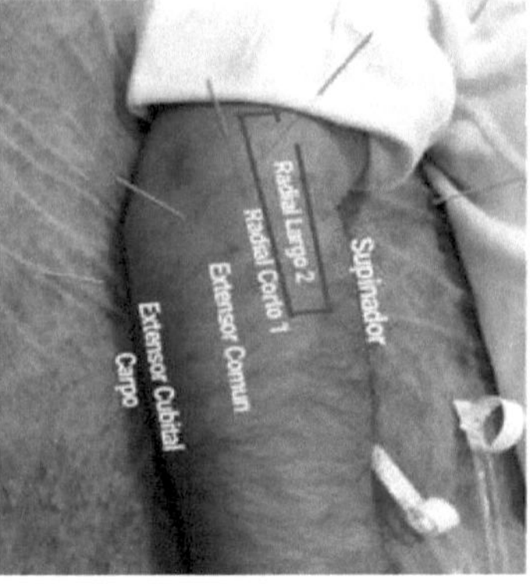

Figure 35. PS in PGM of the extensor carpi radialis longus (40).

- Dangers and precautions: Superficial branch of the radial nerve: Although unlikely to be touched by the needle during the clamp puncture, this nerve runs along the posteromedial aspect of the brachioradialis muscle and lies medial to the extensor carpi radialis longus. However, it is important to be cautious when performing the puncture, following the usual rules to avoid complications (111, 112).

4.4.7. Short radial extensor of the carpus.

- PGMs in the extensor carpi radialis brevis: The PGMs of this muscle are located between the extensor digitorum and extensor carpi radialis longus. With sudden palpation, a local twitch response (REL) can be induced, which facilitates their identification (113, 114).
- Referred pain pattern: The referred pain pattern includes the dorsum of the hand and wrist. However, in the experience of the authors of the text, the most commonly observed pattern includes mainly the epicondylar area, reproducing the characteristic pain of patients with lateral epicondylalgia in 83.3% of cases (113, 114).
- Symptoms: Pain and weakness on grip and extension of the wrist, difficulty flexing the wrist due to stiffness, pain when grasping objects such as glasses, opening doors, or performing any manual grasping movement. In more severe cases, there may be pain at rest (113, 114).
- Trigger mechanisms: Direct trigger mechanisms include repetitive activities that require constant manual force or prolonged pressure, such as factory work, cleaning, or the use of hand tools. Indirect

mechanisms as in the extensor carpi radialis longus, cervical conditions or PGMs in related muscles (such as the brachioradialis, extensor digitorum, and neck and shoulder muscles) may contribute to trigger point activation in this muscle (113, 114).

- Related Muscles: extensor carpi radialis longus, brachioradialis, extensor digitorum, triceps brachii (113, 114).
- PS of the extensor carpi radialis brevis muscle (113, 114):
    - Patient Position: The patient should be supine, with the elbow in slight flexion and the forearm in pronation.
    - Muscle palpation: It is performed just behind the extensor carpi radialis longus, with the aim of provoking a local spasm response (REL) that allows locating the PGM. The trigger point is usually found more caudal than in the extensor carpi radialis longus. The PGM is grasped between the index and middle fingers before inserting the needle.
    - Needle size: A 0.25 mm x 40 mm needle is used to pass through the muscle in the anteroposterior direction.

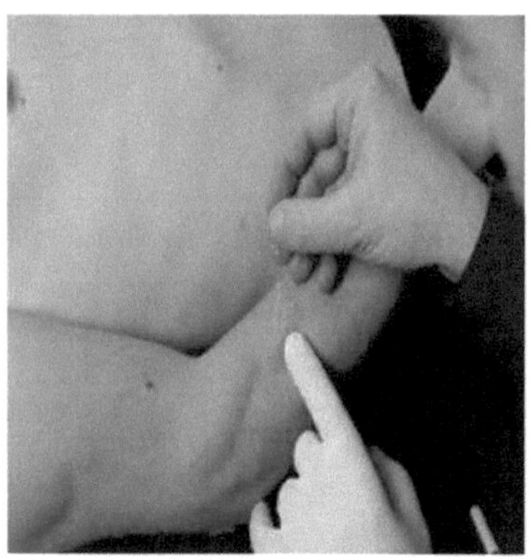

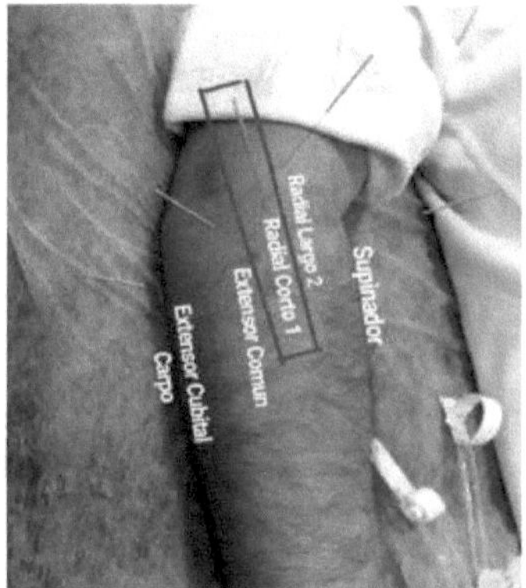

Figure 36. PS in PGM of the extensor carpi radialis brevis (66).

- Dangers and precautions: There is the posterior cutaneous nerve of the forearm that runs above the muscle, so care must be taken to avoid puncturing this nerve. The superficial radial nerve runs beneath the brachioradialis muscle and is distant from the extensor pollicis brevis, making accidental puncture unlikely. However, due to possible anatomical variants, it is recommended to follow the usual precautions when puncturing areas close to nerves (113, 114).

4.4.8. Ulnar extensor of the carpus.

- Location and palpation of the PGMs: The PGMs of the extensor carpi ulnaris muscle are located just proximal to the ulnar border of the extensor digitorum. These trigger points are accessible to flat palpation, a few centimeters below the lateral epicondyle, dorsal to the bony border of the ulna (115, 116).
- Referred pain pattern: The referred pain described includes the ulnar side of the dorsum of the wrist. However, it is noted that it can also be referred to the proximal insertion, affecting the tip and posterior part of the epicondyle, with a pattern similar to that of the anconeus muscle. In these cases, the extensor carpi ulnaris may be involved in rare lateral epicondylalgia, where the pain is located behind the epicondyle (115, 116).
- Clinical symptoms (115, 116):
  - Pain when performing a contraction in shortening, that is, when extending the wrist voluntarily and resisted, especially when associated with ulnar deviation.
  - The most common diagnosis for patients with myofascial pain syndrome (MPS) in this muscle is extensor carpi ulnaris tendinopathy.
- Mechanisms of PGM activation (115, 116):
  - Direct mechanisms: PGMs in this muscle are less frequent and are usually activated due to severe trauma (such as ulnar fractures), elbow surgeries or major overloads in sports such as canoeing or bodybuilding exercises.
  - Indirect mechanisms: Include cervical conditions (herniated disc, joint dysfunctions), PGMs in muscles such as the scalenes, serratus posterosuperior, or adhesive capsulitis.
- Related muscles: radial extensors of the wrist, extensor of the fingers, serratus posterosuperior, scalenes, dry needling of the extensor carpi ulnaris muscle, patient position the patient is placed in the supine position, with the forearm in pronation and the palm of the hand resting on the table, with the elbow slightly flexed (115, 116).
- Palpation of the muscle: Palpate just ulnar to the extensor of the little finger and extensor of the fingers, and dorsal to the bony border of the ulna. It is recommended to locate the ulnar border first and then palpate the muscle immediately behind it (115, 116).

- Needle size: A 0.25 mm x 25 mm needle is used in adults. The muscle is traversed in the direction of the bone and also in the ulnar to radial direction (115, 116).

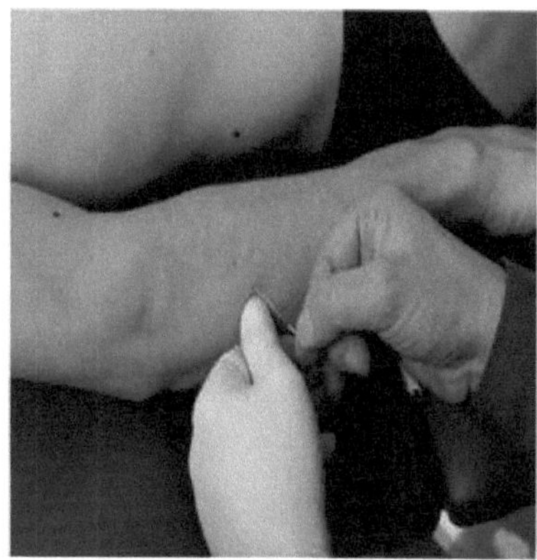

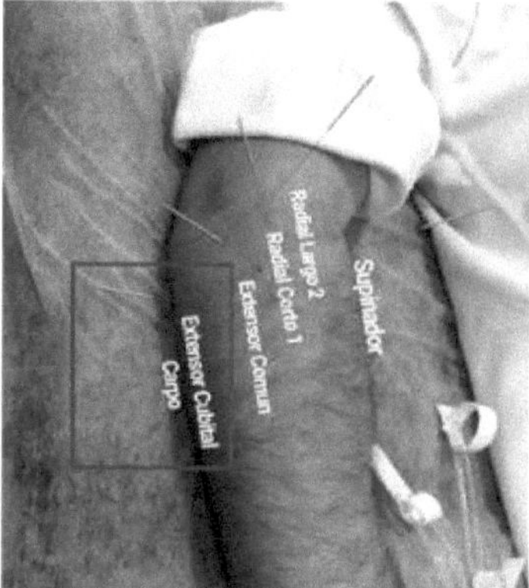

Figure 37. PS in PGM for the extensor carpi ulnaris (66).

- Precautions: Although the radial neurovascular bundle and ulnar nerve are usually beyond the reach of the needle, there is a moderate risk of puncture of the posterior interosseous nerve if the needle reaches the insertion of the supinator muscle. The usual precautions should be taken to avoid this puncture, especially if working near important nerves (115, 116).

4.4.9. Finger extensor and little finger extensor.

- Location and palpation of the PGMs: The PGMs of the extensor digitorum extensor muscle are easily identified by palpation. They are distributed in the fibers corresponding to each finger, and their identification is facilitated by locating the universal tense band corresponding to the third finger (117, 118).
- Referred pain pattern: The referred pain projects along the dorsum of the affected finger, affecting the metacarpophalangeal and proximal interphalangeal joints, but does not reach the last phalanx. The overflow pattern includes the dorsum of the forearm and hand, extending from the PGM to the corresponding finger. For the middle finger, pain may radiate to the ventral aspect of the wrist. PGMs in the fourth and fifth finger fibers may cause pain in the epicondyle,

although according to the authors of the text, this pain may also originate in the middle finger fibers (117, 118).

- Clinical symptoms (117, 118):
  - Pain and stiffness in the affected finger joints, especially the proximal metacarpophalangeal and interphalangeal joints.
  - Sensation of weakness in the grip, mainly if the affected fibers correspond to the third finger.
  - Finger cramps when performing manual activities, such as shaking hands, lifting objects or using the computer keyboard.
  - Pain when performing activities that require a firm grip, with pain at rest and nocturnal pain that awakens the patient in the most severe cases.
- Common associated diagnoses: The patient with PGM in this muscle is often misdiagnosed with lateral epicondylalgia, osteoarthritis or arthritis of the fingers (117, 118).
- Mechanisms of PGM activation (117, 118):
  - Direct mechanisms: These trigger points are activated by energetic overuse of the fingers in activities such as playing the piano, office work (clerical), or repetitive and strong manual presses (tennis players, mechanics, butchers).
  - Indirect mechanisms: They include cervical conditions (herniated disc, cervical joint dysfunctions), the presence of PGMs in neighboring or synergistic muscles, such as the scalenes, serratus posterosuperioris, radial carpal extensors, brachioradialis, triceps brachii and supinator.
- Related muscles: long and short radial extensors of the carpus, brachioradialis, triceps brachii, supinator, scalenes, serratus posterosuperioris, dry needling of the extensor digitorum muscle (117, 118).
- PS (117, 118):
  - Patient position: The patient should be positioned supine, with the forearm in pronation and the hand relaxed. The elbow should be slightly flexed.
  - Identification of the PGMs: The PGMs are located by flat palpation, using the taut band corresponding to the fibers of the third finger as a reference.

- Needle size: A 0.25 mm x 40 mm needle is recommended for puncture, although a 0.25 mm x 25 mm needle can be used in cases of poorly muscled forearms.
- Puncture technique: The puncture should be performed until contacting the radius bone as a reference. This technique allows crossing the posterior part of the supinator muscle, whose PGMs can be found immediately below the extensor digitorum and are relevant in cases of lateral epicondylalgia.

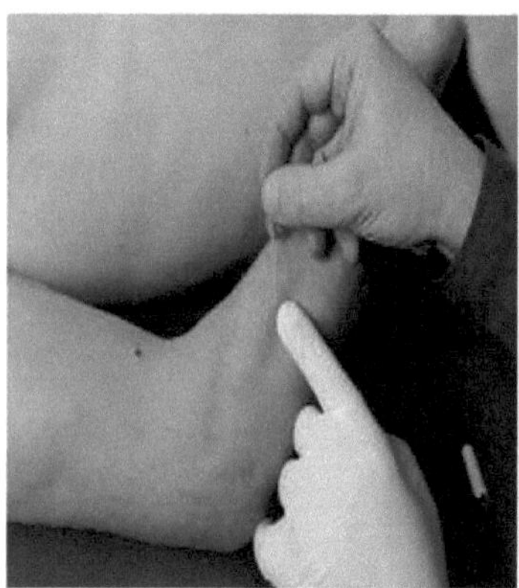

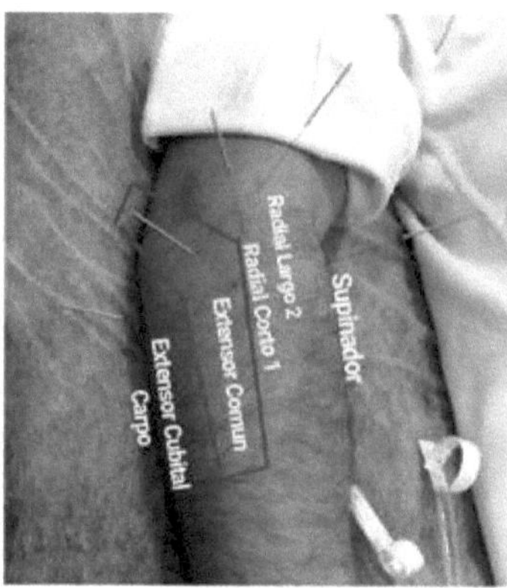

Figure 38. PS in PGM of the extensor digitorum longus (66).

- Precautions: There is a risk of puncture of the posterior interosseous nerve (deep branch of the radial nerve) when crossing the two heads of the supinator muscle. Therefore, the usual precautions should be taken in these cases (117, 118).

4.4.10. Index extender.

- Location and characteristics: The extensor digitorum extensor muscle is located in the distal third of the forearm, between the radius and ulna, and is covered by the tendons of the finger extensors. PGMs are located in the medial part of the muscle belly and refer pain to the radial side of the dorsum of the wrist, especially in the area where its tendon and its myorendinous junction cross the wrist. Generally, the pain does not radiate to the fingers (119, 120).
- Clinical symptoms (119, 120):
  - Pain and stiffness on active extension movements of the wrist and index finger.

- Index extensor PGMs rarely occur in isolation; they are often a painful sequela that persists in the wrist after removal of PGMs in other wrist and finger extensor muscles.

- Related muscles: The PGMs of the index extensor are related to the rest of the extensor muscles of the wrist and fingers (119, 120).
- PS (119, 120):
  - Patient position: The patient is positioned in supine decubitus, with the forearm in pronation and the elbow slightly flexed. The hand should be relaxed and resting on the treatment table.
  - Identification of PGMs: Given their location under the extensor tendons, it can be difficult to identify tight bands. Therefore, look for an exquisitely painful spot in the distal third of the forearm, between the ulna and radius.
  - Puncture technique: It is recommended to use a 0.25 mm x 25 mm needle. The needle is preferably oriented towards the ulna to avoid going too deep through the interosseous membrane.

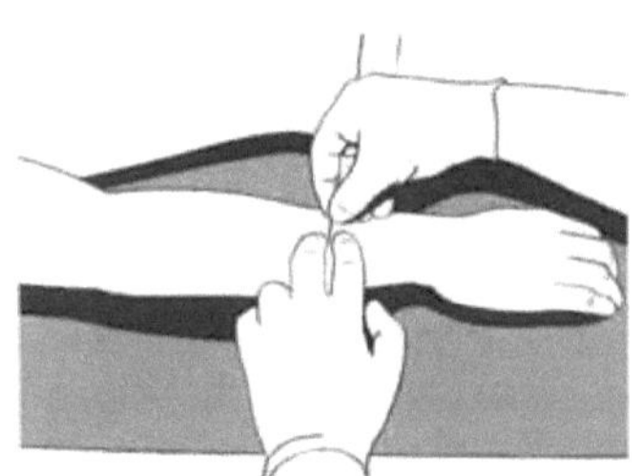
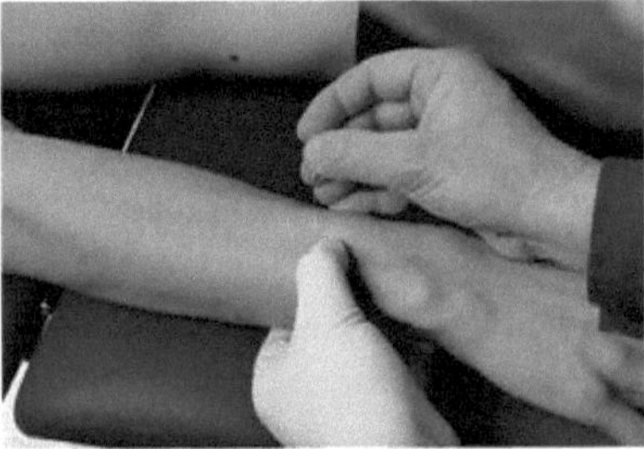

Figure 39. PS in PGM of the index extensor (40, 66).

- Precautions during puncture: There is a very low risk of superficial contact with the medial cutaneous nerve of the forearm, so advance the needle with caution, especially in the first few millimeters of its insertion. At the superficial level, care should also be taken to avoid superficial veins that may be present. Orienting the needle toward the ulna minimizes the risk of crossing the interosseous membrane and contacting the median nerve. However, there is always the possibility of crossing structures such as the anterior and posterior interosseous arteries. Therefore, it is important to maintain good ischemia during puncture and to perform correct hemostasis at the end of the procedure (119, 120).

4.4.11. Supinator.

- Location of the PGMs (121, 122):
  - PGM zones: Two PGM zones are identified in the supinator muscle:
  - Most common area: Located on the anterior aspect of the forearm, near the insertion on the ventral aspect of the radius. This area is accessible to palpation, just next to the insertion of the biceps tendon on the bicipital tuberosity of the radius.
  - Insertional zone: Located on the posterior aspect of the muscle, behind the radius, and covered by the extensor carpi ulnaris and extensor digitorum muscles, which makes direct palpation difficult.
- Referred pain: The most common pain pattern associated with the supinator muscle is described as pain radiating to the lateral epicondyle and its surroundings, both anteriorly and posteriorly, as well as to the dorsal side of the first interdigital commissure. Although this muscle is considered to contribute to lateral epicondylalgia, the clinical experience of the authors of this text suggests that its involvement is not as prevalent as has been claimed, with one study indicating a 50% involvement rate in patients diagnosed with lateral epicondylar enthesopathy (121, 122).
- Activation mechanisms: The PGMs of the supinator muscle can be activated during activities involving forceful supinations of the elbow, such as playing tennis, carrying suitcases, or any action requiring significant elbow stress with the forearm in pronation (e.g., opening jars, shaking hands). Pain may persist even at rest after activation (121, 122).
- Clinical symptoms: epicondylar pain that manifests during vigorous contractions of the muscle, which remains present even at rest (121, 122).
- Related muscles: radial extensors of the carpus, brachioradialis, extensor digitorum, brachialis, triceps, biceps brachii, and palmaris longus (121, 122).
- PS (121, 122):
  - Patient Position: The patient is placed in supine decubitus, with the elbow extended and the forearm in supination.
  - Location of the PGM: The muscle is palpated just lateral to the insertion of the biceps brachii tendon at the tuberosity of the

radius, separating out the muscle mass of the extensor carpi radialis longus and brachioradialis.

- Puncture Technique: Although it may be difficult to locate due to its depth, a painful nodule is usually perceived when pressing longitudinally towards the radius. Once located, the PGM is fixed between the fingers against the radius and punctured with a 0.25 mm x 40 mm needle looking for contact with the radius as a reference.
- Options for Locating the PGM
  - Option 1: Include lateral tilts of the needle to grope in the direction of the radius, allowing traversing the part of the muscle most likely to contain the PGM.
  - Option 2: Maintain the anteroposterior direction of the needle while asking the patient to perform millimetric pronation movements, which helps to access the lateral areas of the supinator muscle, which is slightly stretched during rotation.
  - Recommendation: Opting for the second option reduces the risk of puncture of the lateral cutaneous nerve of the forearm compared to the first option.

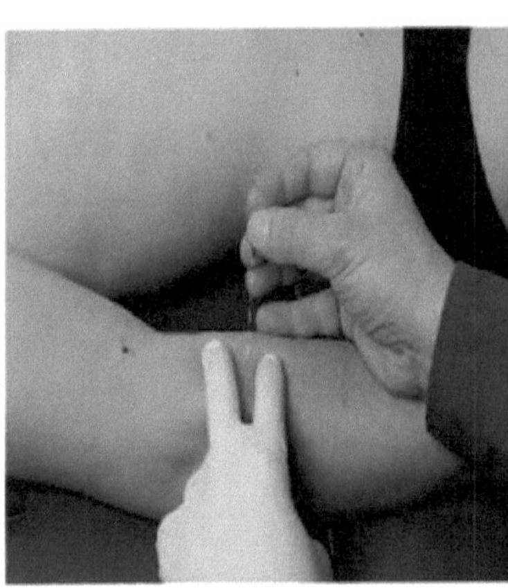

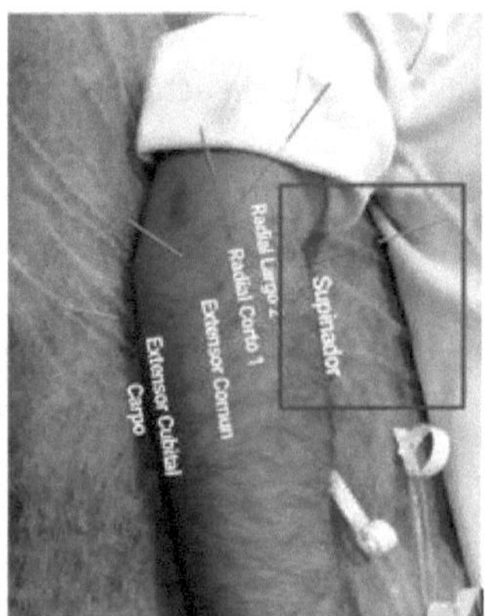

Figure 40. PS in PGM of the supinator (66).

- Dangers and precautions: Puncture of the supinator muscle presents the risk of affecting the posterior interosseous nerve (deep branch of the radial nerve). During puncture of the anterior areas, there is also a risk of contacting the lateral cutaneous nerve of the forearm and the superficial radial nerve. If the needle is directed too medially, there may also be a risk of affecting the median nerve (121, 122).

4.4.12. Round pronator.

- PGM localization: The pronator teres is a muscle of the volar aspect of the forearm characterized by its penniform architecture. The ratio of the length of its fibers to the total length of the muscle is low, which makes it difficult to identify tight bands, although it is easier to locate sensitive areas that indicate the presence of MMPs at different heights of the muscle (123, 124).
- Referred pain pattern: According to Simons et al, the referred pain pattern of pronator teres extends along the radial area of the anterior aspect of the wrist and forearm. However, the authors' clinical experience suggests that the most common pattern is located in the insertion zone of the muscle at the epitrochlea, being responsible for pain at this level along with other muscles such as the triceps and pectoralis major (123, 124).
- Clinical symptoms: Patients with PGM in the pronator teres have difficulty supinating the hand with the elbow extended (123, 124).
- Activation mechanisms (123, 124):
  - Mechanical overloads: PGMs can be activated by overloads related to pronation and flexion actions of the elbow, typically seen in sports such as tennis.
  - Trauma: Injuries such as elbow fractures (especially of the radial head) or wrist fractures are frequent causes of PGM activation in this muscle.
  - Pathological conditions: PGMs have also been identified in the pronator teres related to superficial lymphatic thrombosis, especially in patients who have undergone lymphadenectomy for breast cancer.
  - Relationship with other muscles: The location of the pronator teres roundus in the referred pain zone of other muscles such as the pectoralis major and minor and triceps brachii may be a cause of activation and perpetuation of their PGMs.
- PS (123, 124):
  - Patient position: The patient should be positioned in supine decubitus with the forearm in supination.
  - PGM location: Locate the PGM and fix it between the fingers.

- Puncture technique: A 0.25 mm x 25 mm needle is used for thin forearms, or 0.30 mm x 40 mm for larger forearms.

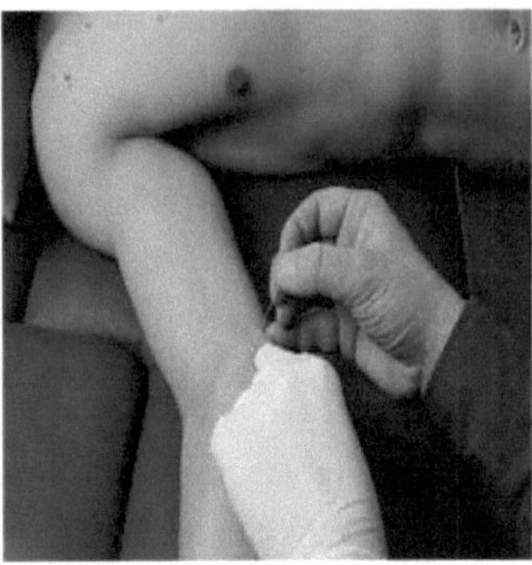

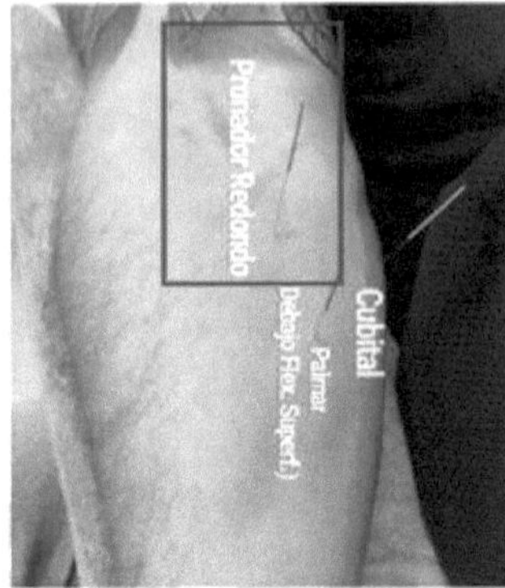

Figure 41. PS in PGM of the pronator teres roundus (66).

- Dangers and precautions: Risk of puncture of the median nerve, this nerve passes between the two heads of the pronator teres muscle. To avoid accidental puncture. It is essential to be attentive to the needle location to prevent complications (123, 124).

4.4.13. Ulnar flexor carpi ulnaris.

- Anatomy and location of MMPs: The flexor carpi ulnaris has a bipenniform structure, which allows its innervation band to run longitudinally. This means that the PGMs can be located at any height of the muscle, including areas close to the myorendinous junction zones (125, 126).
- Referred pain pattern: The referred pain is projected over the area where the tendon of the muscle crosses the wrist and at its insertion in the pisiform. This pattern is reproduced during contraction of the muscle, specifically when performing flexion with ulnar tilt. This makes the most likely diagnosis in these cases to be carpal ulnar flexor tendinopathy (125, 126).
- Relationship with other muscles: It has been observed that the PGMs of this muscle can be related to pain in the epitrochlear area. However, it is not clear whether this represents a different pain pattern or whether it is a pain related to insertional PGMs. Activation of PGMs may be caused by (125, 126):

- Direct mechanisms: Mechanical overload, such as from performing certain movements.
- Indirect mechanisms: PGM activation of other muscles such as pectoralis minor, latissimus dorsi, or serratus posterosuperioris.

- PS (125, 126):
  - Patient Position: The patient should be supine with the shoulder in slight abduction and external rotation, as well as having the elbow extended.
  - Location of the PGM: The PGM must be located and fixed for the puncture.
  - Puncture technique: A 0.25 mm x 40 mm needle is used, directed towards the PGM.

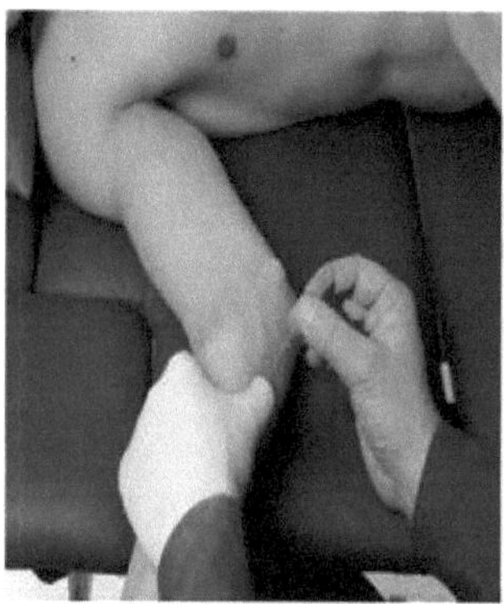

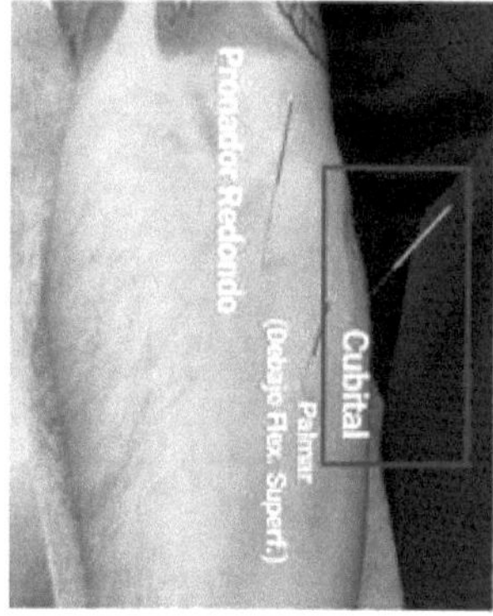

Figure 42. PS in PGM of the flexor carpi ulnaris (66).

- Dangers and precautions: Risk of ulnar nerve puncture: this nerve passes close to the ulnar flexor carpi ulnaris. Maintaining a careful approach to the puncture technique is vital to prevent complications (125, 126).

4.4.14. Radial flexor of the carpus.

- Referred pain pattern: radial carpal flexor carpal PGMs report pain in the area where their tendon crosses the wrist, particularly in the volar and radial areas of the wrist. This pain tends to appear during active wrist flexion movements, which frequently leads to a diagnosis of wrist tendinitis (127, 128).

- Functional difficulties: Patients with PGM in this muscle may experience problems when using tools such as large scissors or shears, commonly used in gardening (127, 128).
- Palpation and localization: Palpation of the radial flexor carpi radialis PGMs is relatively straightforward. Although it can be difficult to identify structures on the volar aspect of the forearm, this muscle is easily located using the pronator teres as a reference, since it is located subcutaneously and on the ulnar side of it (127, 128).
- Activation of PGMs (127, 128):
  - Direct causes: PGMs can be triggered by:
    - Overloads related to gripping thin tools (e.g., carpentry tools).
    - Use of ski or golf clubs.
    - More severe trauma, such as an elbow fracture.
  - Indirect causes: Activation may also be due to key PGMs in other muscles, such as the pectoralis minor or in muscles that include the area of referred pain, such as the serratus anterior or triceps brachii. This is especially relevant when there are biomechanical links with other muscles, such as pronator teres and palmaris longus.
- PS (127, 128):
  - Patient Position: The patient should be supine with the elbow extended and the forearm supinated.
  - PGM localization: The PGMs of the muscle are palpated and fixed for puncture.
  - Puncture technique: A needle of 0.25 mm x 25 mm or larger is used, depending on the thickness of the forearm.

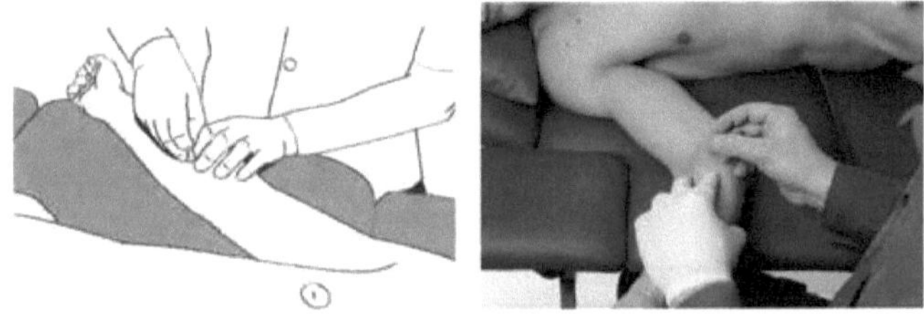

Figure 43. PS in PGM of the radial carpal flexor (40, 66).

- Hazards and precautions (127, 128):

- Risk of nerve puncture: There is a risk of the needle contacting branches of the medial and lateral cutaneous nerves of the forearm. Therefore, it is crucial to introduce the needle slowly, especially in the first few millimeters of penetration.
- Median nerve: There is also a possibility of contact with the median nerve if the needle is inserted too far or directed too laterally.

4.4.15. Long palmar.

- Anatomy and Location of the PGMs: The PGM of the palmaris longus muscle is easy to locate as it is located in the most superficial plane, just medial to the radial flexor carpi radialis and lateral to the flexor carpi ulnaris (129, 130).
- Referred pain pattern: According to Simons et al. the most common pain pattern associated with palmar palmaris longus manifests as superficial itching or prickling in the palm of the hand, as well as pain in the center of the palm. This pain extends towards the base of the thumb and the distal ridge of the palm, without reaching the fingers (129, 130).
- Additional symptoms: Patients with PGM in the palmaris longus have pain, weakness and hypersensitivity in the palm of the hand when performing manual grasping activities, such as handling tools (129, 130).
- Mechanisms of PGM activation: Although the palmaris longus muscle may present different activation mechanisms, it has been observed that the presence of PGMs in neighboring muscles, such as the triceps brachii (in its medial belly), may be related both to PGM activation in the palmaris longus and to their perpetuation (129, 130).
- PS (129, 130):
  - Patient position: The patient should be supine, with the elbow extended and the forearm supinated, and the palm of the hand facing upward.
  - Location of the PGM: The muscle is palpated just medial to the belly of the flexor carpi radialis and lateral to the belly of the flexor carpi ulnaris. The PGM is easy to identify by pressing against the ulna.
  - Puncture technique: A 0.25 mm x 25 mm needle is used for the puncture, similar to that described for the radial carpal flexor.

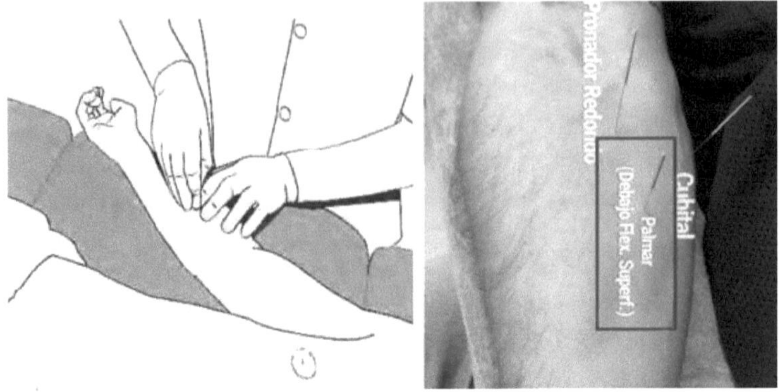

Figure 44. PS in PGM of the long palmar (40).

- Hazards and precautions (129, 130):
  - Risk of nerve puncture: Superficially, there is a risk of the needle contacting branches of the medial cutaneous nerve of the forearm. Therefore, it is important to introduce the needle slowly to avoid complications.
  - Ulnar nerve: There is also a possibility of contact with the ulnar nerve if the needle is too deep and too medially inclined.

4.4.16. Common superficial and deep flexors of the fingers and flexor digitorum longus of the thumb.

- Anatomy and referred pain (131, 132):
  - Both superficial flexor and deep flexor fingers present a similar referred pain pattern. This pain manifests in the corresponding finger where the fibers containing the PGMs act, often radiating to the elbow on its palmar aspect.
  - Pain sensation: The pain can be described as a "lightning" sensation radiating to the affected finger. According to Kellgren, the common flexor digitorum profundus can cause "joint" pain in the metacarpophalangeal joints.
  - Thumb flexor pollicis longus: PGMs of the thumb flexor pollicis longus cause similar pain, extending along the anterior aspect of the thumb to the tip of its distal phalanx.
- Clinical difficulties (131, 132):

- Identification: Due to the deep location of the PGMs in these muscles, they are not directly palpable, and taut bands cannot be identified. The suspicion of PGMs is based on the clinical presentation of the patient, who may experience pain and difficulty when using tools that require forceps or digital grasping, such as scissors.
- Mobility restriction: One way to assess function is to ask the patient to place the palms of the hands facing each other, with the palmar sides of the fingers well glued together. When performing extension of both wrists, if the fibers of any finger flexor harbor PGM, the corresponding finger will not be able to stay glued to its counterpart on the other hand, tending to flex. This occurs because finger extension competes with wrist extension.

- Symptoms (131, 132):
  - Pain: Localized in the affected fingers, with possible "lightning" sensations.
  - Weakness: In finger grasping movements, which may affect daily activities.
- PS (131, 132):
  - Lancing Technique: Puncture of the PGMs in the common flexor digitorum and flexor pollicis longus muscles is performed similarly to the technique used for palmaris longus and flexor carpi radialis, but using a 0.25 mm x 40 mm or 0.30 mm x 50 mm needle.
  - Patient Position: The patient should be in supine decubitus, with the forearm supinated and the elbow extended, to facilitate localization of the PGMs.

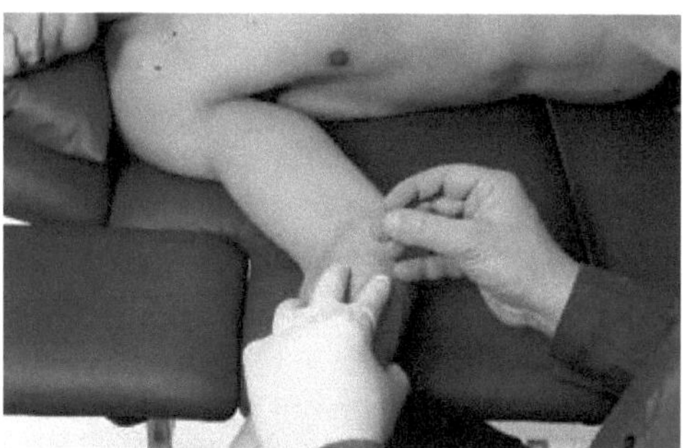

PS in PGM for superficial and deep common flexors of the fingers and long flexor of the thumb (66).

- Hazards and precautions (131, 132):
    - Risk of nerve puncture: Depending on the location of the PGM, there is a risk of the needle contacting the median nerve or ulnar nerve. This, combined with the type of "flashing" pain that these PGMs sometimes cause, may raise doubts as to whether a PGM or a nerve has been touched.
    - Ultrasound-guided: Ultrasound-guided puncture could be considered to avoid neurovascular structures, especially if safety cannot be guaranteed during puncture.
    - Prevention rules: If ultrasound is not used, it is crucial to follow the prevention rules to avoid nerve puncture by keeping the fingers of the hand free to move in case a "lightning" response (REL) occurs. This will help decide whether the needle has touched a nerve or a PGM.

4.4.17. Square pronator.

- Context and symptoms: The literature has not extensively documented the existence of PGM in pronator quadratus, but a study by Hwang et al. investigated the referred symptoms of this muscle in a sample of 35 healthy men. These patients received intramuscular injections of hypertonic saline (0.3 ml 16%) guided by electromyography. The results showed two predominant patterns of referred pain (133, 134):
    - Pattern 1: Described by 57% of the subjects, it extended along the ulnar border of the forearm and hand, reaching in some cases the medial epicondyle and the fifth finger. The most intense pain was experienced at the base of the fifth finger.
    - Pattern 2: Described by 29% of the subjects, it was mainly projected distally, covering the third and fourth fingers, with the most intense pain in the middle part of the distal portion of the forearm, both dorsal and volar.
    - All participants in the study rated their pain at a level of 9 out of 10 or higher, describing it as deep, diffuse and throbbing. Some also reported numbness or tingling in the affected area.
- Activation mechanisms: The pronator quadratus may be activated by daily or work activities involving overload, such as wringing clothes or loosening screws. It is suggested that if a patient presents with activation of a PGM in this muscle, symptoms are likely to be similar

to those described above. We reported a successful case of diagnosis and treatment of a PGM in pronator quadratus in a patient with wrist and hand pain following a consolidated wrist fracture. We recommend including pronator quadratus PGMs in the differential diagnosis of patients with pain in the distribution of the C7-C8 dermatomes or areas innervated by the median and ulnar nerves, especially in the absence of neurologic pathology (133, 134).

- PS (133, 134):
  - Puncture Technique: Due to the location of the pronator quadratus, which is volar but closer to the dorsal side, it is recommended to perform the puncture from the dorsal side, where there are fewer neurovascular structures.
  - To find the PGM, it is recommended to palpate alternately on both sides of the forearm until a painful point that reproduces the patient's pain is located. The puncture is performed using a 0.25 mm x 40 mm needle, penetrating up to approximately 25 mm in a dorsovolar direction.
  - Patient Position: The patient should be supine, with the forearm in pronation.
  - Needle Guidance: Advance the needle until you feel that the interosseous membrane has been crossed, which occurs before crossing the deep part of the muscle.

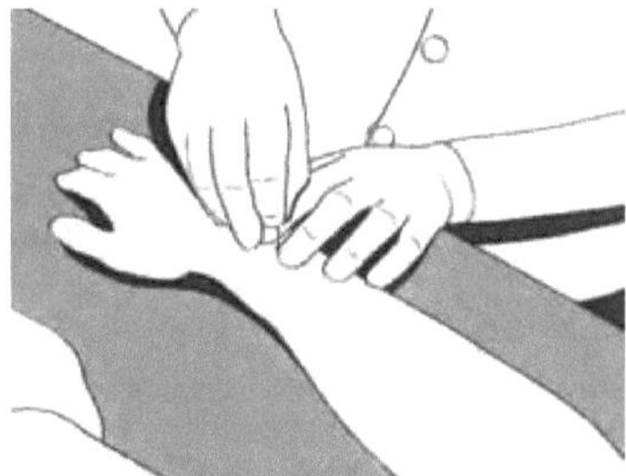

Figure 46. PS in PGM for square pronator (40).

- Dangers and Precautions: The main danger lies in the potential for damage to neurovascular structures. Although these structures are generally located anterior to the pronator quadratus, there is a risk of contact with the ulnar nerve or median nerve if the needle is inserted too deep or angled in inappropriate directions. For added safety, electromyography-guided puncture can be performed. It is essential to follow precautionary rules to avoid puncturing a nerve, and to take special care when advancing the needle in the first few millimeters to avoid the dorsal cutaneous nerve of the forearm (133, 134).

4.4.18. Eminence tenar.

- Context and symptoms: Although PGMs have not been described in the abductor pollicis brevis of the thumb, they have been identified in other muscles of the tenar eminence, such as the adductor pollicis, opponens pollicis and flexor pollicis brevis. The most common referred pain patterns are (134, 135):
- Adductor Thumb: Pain is localized on the external aspect of the thumb and at the base of the thumb. It may extend to the palmar surface of the first metacarpophalangeal joint, the elbow of the thumb, the tenar eminence and the dorsal aspect of the first interdigital space.
- Thumb Opponent: Pain manifests on the palmar surface of most of the thumb and in a small area on the radial side of the volar aspect of the wrist.
- Activation mechanisms: Pain in these muscles may occur when performing tasks that require precise manipulation, such as writing, putting on clothing, or fastening a button. It is also common for patients to report a feeling of weakness in activities that demand the prehensile grip of the thumb. In addition, the presence of PGMs in related muscles such as the supinator, extensor carpi radialis longus, brachioradialis, brachioradialis and scalenes may generate pain referred to the first interdigital space, suggesting the need to include these muscles in treatment (134, 135).
- PS of the muscles of the tenar eminence (134, 135):
    - Adductor of the thumb:
        - Patient Position: Supine decubitus with the elbow slightly flexed and the forearm in pronation.
        - Palpation: Locate the muscle in pincer with the thumb on the dorsal aspect of the first interdigita space.
        - Needle: A 0.16 mm x 25 mm needle is recommended, which is introduced from the dorsal side of the hand, crossing if necessary the first dorsal interosseous and directing it towards the adjacent finger.

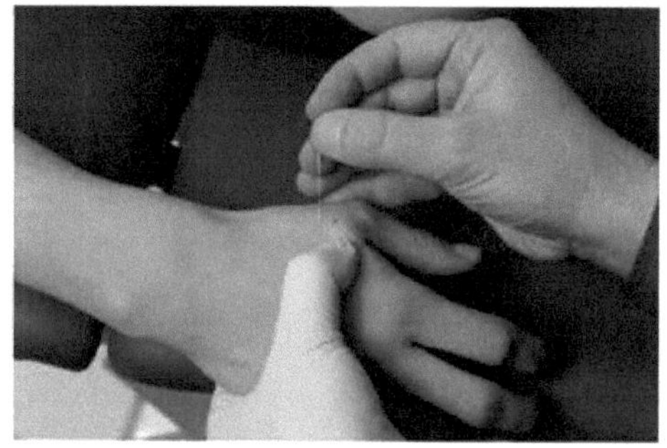

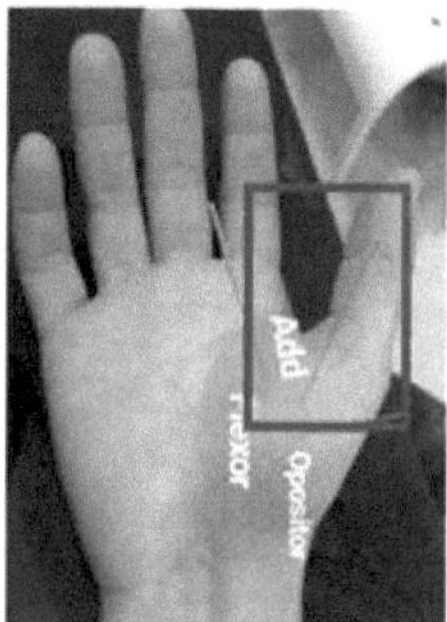

Figure 47. PS in PGM of the thumb adductor (66).

- Opponent of the thumb:
  - Patient Position: Supine decubitus with the elbow extended and the forearm supinated.
  - Needle: Use a 0.16 mm x 25 mm needle, directing it in an anteroposterior direction towards the PGM. Make sure that the palpating hand does not impede the opposing movement of the thumb, looking for bone contact to confirm that the muscle has been crossed.

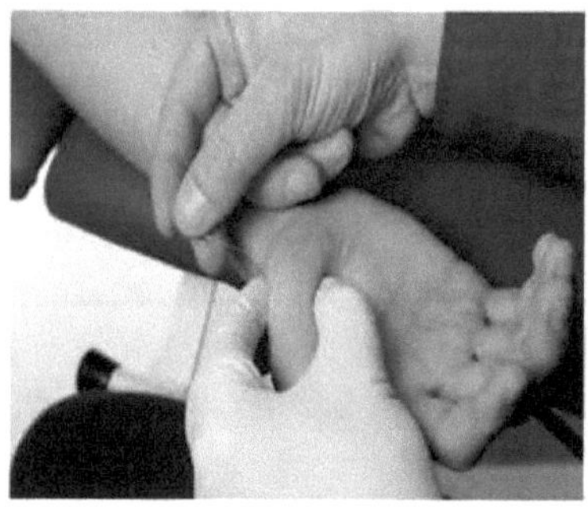

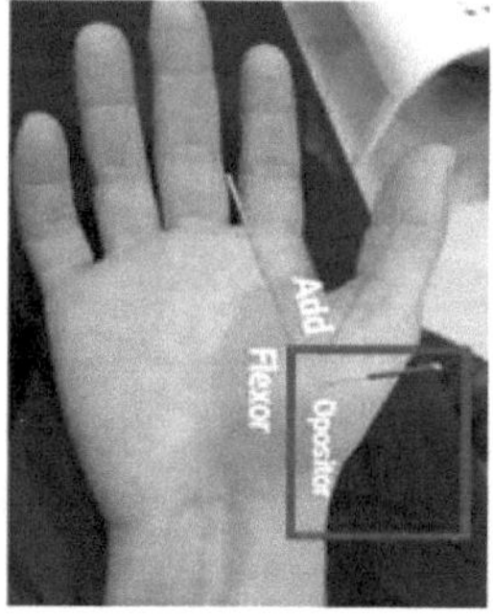

Figure 48. PS in PGM of the thumb opponent (66).

- Flexor digitorum brevis of the thumb:
  - Patient Position: Same as for the opponent.
  - Palpation: Identify the flexor pollicis longus tendon by palpating the sides of the thumb for a sore spot, usually located radially to the tendon.
  - Needle: A 0.16 mm x 25 mm needle is introduced into the PGM.

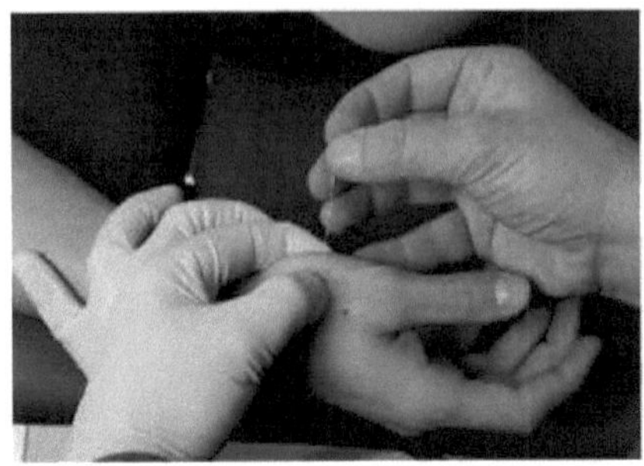

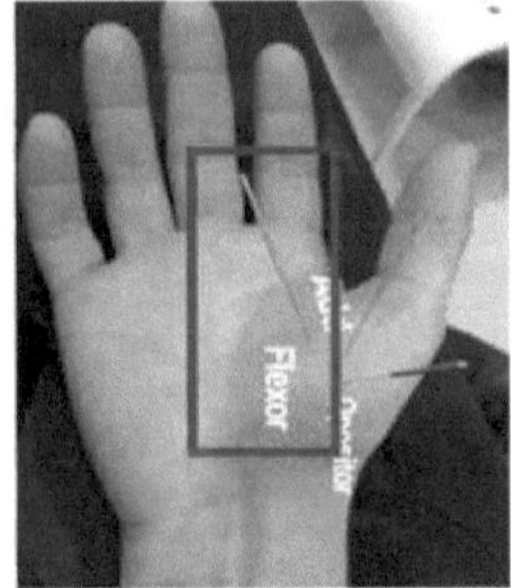

Figure 49. PS in PGM of the short flexor of the thumb (66).

- Hazards and precautions (134, 135):
  - Vascular Risks: Branches of the radial artery and the cephalic vein are present in the tenar eminence. Puncture of these vessels may cause stabbing pain and excessive bleeding, so adequate compression should be performed during puncture and proper hemostasis should be ensured.
  - Neurological risks: The deep motor branch of the ulnar nerve and the common palmar digital nerves may be affected, so it is crucial to take adequate precautions when performing the puncture.

4.4.19. Hypotenar eminence.

- Symptoms and referred pain: The referred pain pattern of the little finger abductor muscle extends along the ulnar border of the fifth finger, reaching the distal interphalangeal joint. This pattern is similar to the pain elicited by the interosseous muscles. The presence of PGMs in this muscle is associated with Heberden's nodes in the distal interphalangeal joint, as well as hyperalgesia (increased pain sensitivity) in that area. Although no trigger points have been described in the flexor pollicis brevis or opponens of the little finger, it is possible that these muscles are related to pain in the hypothenar eminence, the fifth metacarpal and the little finger itself (136, 137).
- PS: Dry needling of the little finger abductor can be performed in two ways, depending on how the trigger point was located during palpation (136, 137):
  - Flat:

    - Palpation: The muscle is pressed against the ulnar border of the metacarpal bone.
    - Needle: A 0.16 mm x 25 mm needle is used, which is inserted towards the bone. The patient's hand should be supinated (palm up).
- Clamped:
    - Palpation: The muscle is grasped in forceps.
    - Needle: It is inserted through the dorsal side of the hand, also with a 0.16 mm x 25 mm needle. The patient's hand should be in pronation (palm down).

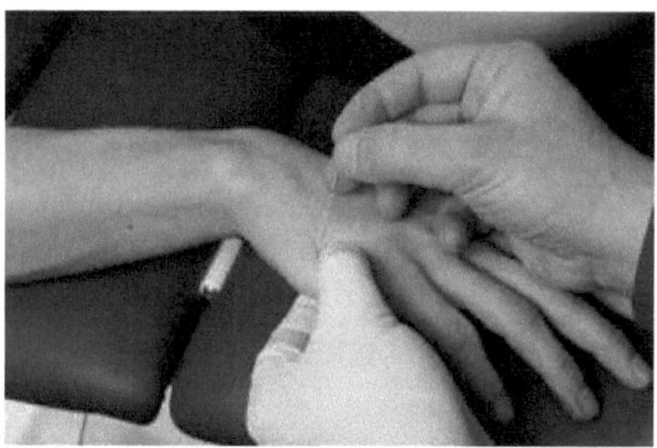

PS for PGM in abductor of the little finger (66).

- Dangers and precautions: Since several nerve branches pass through the area, both cutaneous (palmar branch of the ulnar nerve, common and proper palmar digital nerves) and muscular (superficial and deep branches of the ulnar nerve), it is essential to follow the precautions indicated in the safety protocols to avoid injury to these structures (136, 137).

4.4.20. Interosseous and lumbricals of the little finger.

- Symptoms and referred pain: The pattern of referred pain from the dorsal and palmar interossei is projected towards the finger where the affected muscle inserts, concentrating particularly in the distal interphalangeal joint of that finger. A clear differentiation between dorsal, palmar and lumbrical interosseous referred pain has not yet been established. The pain pattern of the first dorsal interosseous includes a deep pain component in the dorsum of the hand that may extend into the palm and even affect the dorsal aspect of the fifth finger. PGMs in these muscles have been linked to the presence of

Heberden's nodes in the distal interphalangeal joints and hyperalgesia in those areas. It has been observed that treatment of PGMs can reduce joint pain and, in some cases, even decrease the size of the nodules. However, this relationship needs more rigorous studies to be verified. A frequent interrelationship between hand osteoarthritis and interosseous and lumbrical PGMs has also been reported, noting that altered hand biomechanics due to osteoarthritis can cause PGMs, and these in turn aggravate the osteoarthritic condition. Patients with PGMs in these muscles often present with pain, stiffness and weakness in the hands, making it difficult to perform activities such as writing, dressing or manual tasks. Professions that require precision with the hands, such as sewing, painting, or mechanics, may act as triggers for MMPs (136, 137).

- PS (136, 137):
  - Puncture of the interosseous:
    - Patient position: supine decubitus, with the elbow extended and the forearm in pronation.
    - The therapist's palpating hand holds the patient's hand to facilitate finger movement, allowing the identification of the local spasm response (REL) that will indicate the presence of a PGM in the dorsal interosseous or palmar interosseous. The needle used is 0.16 mm x 25 mm, inserted from the back of the hand in the direction of the affected finger.
    - In the case of the first interosseous space, the muscle is palpated with the thumb on the dorsum and the index finger on the palm, directing the needle towards the area of hyperalgesia.
  - Puncture of the lumbricals:
    - Patient position: supine decubitus with the hand in supination. The needle is introduced through the palmar side of the hand, with the therapist's thumb palpating the muscle.
    - If the patient's skin permits, a 0.16 mm x 25 mm needle is used, although if the skin is harder, a thicker 0.25 mm x 25 mm needle may be necessary, which increases discomfort due to the high skin sensitivity in that area. Depending on the patient's tolerance, topical anesthesia or cold may be used to reduce pain.

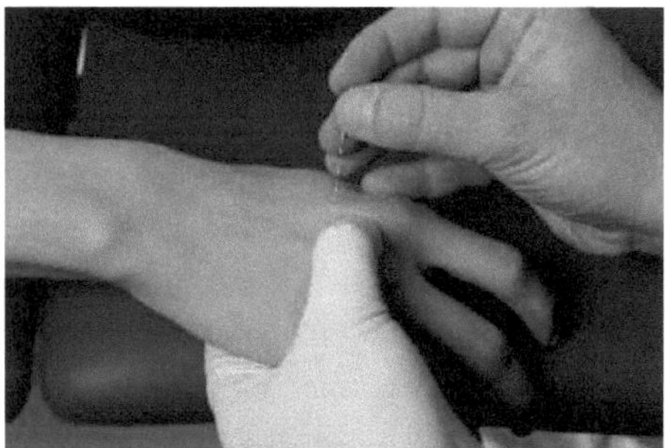

Figure 51. PS in PGM for interosseous and lumbricals of the little finger (66).

- Hazards and precautions (136, 137):
    - Interosseous: Caution should be taken with the nerve and vascular structures that pass through the area, such as the common palmar digital nerves (from the median and ulnar nerves), and the dorsal digital nerves (from the radial and ulnar nerves), as well as the arterial branches of the radial and ulnar arteries, and the dorsal and palmar metacarpal veins. Puncturing a vessel may increase post-puncture pain if adequate hemostasis is not performed.
    - Lumbricals: The main risk is skin sensitivity in the palmar area, which can make the technique more painful. The application of cold or local anesthesia may improve patient tolerance.

Dry needling has proven to be an effective therapeutic technique in the treatment of myofascial trigger points (MTrPs) in the upper limbs, providing considerable pain relief and improving the functionality of the affected muscles. Its application in muscles such as the trapezius, supraspinatus, rhomboids, and the flexors and extensors of the forearm, shows its versatility and efficacy in the treatment of various pathologies. Clinical studies indicate that dry needling not only reduces localized pain, but also improves joint mobility and relieves referred pain in nearby structures.

Direct stimulation of the PGMs in the upper limb facilitates desensitization of hypersensitive areas, improving motor function and reducing disability. However, it is crucial that the physical therapist has adequate training to perform the technique, minimizing risks such as damage to nerve and vascular structures or pneumothorax in delicate areas such as the thorax and shoulder. In addition, more research is needed to further investigate the mechanisms of action and the effectiveness of specific protocols for different populations.

In conclusion, dry needling of the upper limbs is a valuable tool in physiotherapeutic treatment, aiding in pain management and functional recovery. Its integration into a comprehensive therapeutic approach can enhance clinical outcomes and improve the quality of life of patients with musculoskeletal conditions.

BIBLIOGRAPHIC REFERENCES.

1. Simons, D.G., Travell, J.G., Simons, L.S. (2002). Myofascial pain and dysfunction: The trigger point manual. Upper half of the body, 2ed. Madrid: Editorial Médica Panamericana. ISBN: 9788479035754.
2. Dommerholt, J., Fernandez, C. (2018). Trigger Point Dry Needling: An Evidenced and Clinical-Based Approach. 2nd edition. Elselvier. ISBN: 978-0702074165.
3. American Physical Therapy Association (APTA). (2012). Physical therapists and the performance of dry needling. 1-141.
4. Baldry, P. (2005). Acupuncture, trigger points and musculoskeletal pain. 3rd ed. Churchill Livingstone. ISBN: 978-0443066443.
5. Hong, C.Z. (1994). Lidocaine injection versus dry needling to myofascial trigger points: The importance of the local twitch response. American Journal of Physical Medicine and Rehabilitation. 73(4): 256-263.
6. Cummings, T.M., White, A.R. (2001). Needling therapies in the management of myofascial trigger point pain: A systematic review. Archives of Physical Medicine and Rehabilitation. 82(7): 986-992.
7. Tough, E.A., White, A.R., Cummings, T.M., Richards, S.H., Campbell, J.L. (2009). Acupuncture and dry needling in the management of myofascial trigger point pain: A systematic review and meta-analysis of randomized controlled trials. European Journal of Pain. 13(1): 3-10.
8. Kietrys, D.M., Palombaro, K.M., Azzaretto, E. (2013). Effectiveness of dry needling for upper-quarter myofascial pain: A systematic review and meta-analysis. Journal of Orthopaedic and Sports Physical Therapy, 43(9): 620-634.
9. Peuker, E.T., White, A. (1999). Anatomy for the clinical practice of acupuncture. Clinical Anatomy. 12(3): 174-182.
10. Ernst, E., White, A.R. (2001). Prospective studies of the safety of acupuncture: A systematic review. American Journal of Medicine. 110(6): 481-485.
11. Cummings, T.M., Baldry, P. (2007). Regional myofascial pain: Diagnosis and management. Best Practice and Research Clinical Rheumatology. 21(2): 367-387.
12. Aldlyami, E., Kulkarni, A., Reed, M.R., Muller, S.D. (2010). Partington Latex-free gloves: safer for whom? J. Arthroplasty. 25: 27-30.

13. Mayoral, O. (2009). Trigger point dry needling: A simple technique for the treatment of myofascial pain. Fisioterapia. 31(3): 126-134.
14. Ernst, E., White, A. (2001). Acupuncture and dry needling safety review: Infection risks and prevention. American Journal of Medicine. 110(6): 481-485.
15. Peuker, E.T., White, A. (1999). Anatomical considerations and needle safety in acupuncture. Clinical Anatomy. 12(3): 174-182.
16. Dann, J.J., Eckstein, M. (1992). The occurrence of infections with skin punctures: A prospective study of 5,000 punctures without skin preparation. Journal of Clinical Medicine. 8(4): 405-411.
17. Wit, M.J., Johnson, L.C., Baker, S.J. (1997). Risk of infections in trigger point dry needling: A review of 230,000 cases. Acupuncture in Medicine. 15(1): 35-40.
18. Zhang, X., Li, J., Zhou, Q. (2009). Infections in acupuncture and dry needling: Bacterial and viral complications. Chinese Journal of Traditional Medicine. 15(3): 21-28.
19. Rosenblatt, M.A., Abelson, S.A. (2005). Complications and safety considerations in acupuncture and dry needling: Puncture accidents and risk management. Pain Medicine. 6(1): 53-59.
20. García, M. J., López, R. A. (2022). Dry needling considerations: contraindications and precautions. Journal of Physical Therapy and Rehabilitation. 34(2): 123-130.
21. Fernandez, A. L., Torres, S. (2021). Effects of dry needling in patients with complex medical conditions. Journal of Pain Management. 29(4): 45-54.
22. Martinez, P. (2020). Manual therapy and dry needling: a practical guide for the physical therapist. Editorial Médica Panamericana.
23. Sanchez, T., Ruiz, J. (2019). Physical therapy and pain management: contemporary approaches. Elsevier.
24. Perez, L. (2020). Contraindications in dry needling therapy. Advances in physiotherapy. Springer. 245-260.
25. Morales, E. (2018). Assessment and risks in dry needling. In S. Fernandez (Ed.), Contemporary therapies in chronic pain. Editorial Médica. 115-130.
26. Rodriguez, A. (2021). Evaluation of the effectiveness and safety of dry needling in patients with muscle pain: a clinical study. Master's thesis, University of Barcelona.

27. Boyce, J.M., Pittet, D. (2002). Guideline for hand hygiene in health-care settings: Recommendations of the Healthcare Infection Control Practices Advisory Committee and the HICPAC/SHEA/APIC/IDSA Hand Hygiene Task Force. American Journal of Infection Control 30(8): S1-S46.
28. Health Service Executive (HSE). (2009). Standard precautions in health care. Health protection surveillance centre.
29. Strategy for the Control of Antimicrobial Resistance in Ireland (SARI). (2005). Guidelines for hand hygiene in Irish healthcare settings.
30. Ehrenkranz, N.J., Alfonso, B.C. (1991). Failure of bland soap handwash to prevent hand transfer of patient bacteria to urethral catheters. Infection Control and Hospital Epidemiology. 12(11): 654-662.
31. Paulson, D.S., Riccelli, E., Fendler, E. (1999). A comparison of the antimicrobial activity of plain soap, antimicrobial soap, and an alcoholic hand gel. Infection Control and Hospital Epidemiology. 20(6): 396-401.
32. Center for Disease Control and Prevention (CDC). (2019). Guideline for infection control in healthcare personnel. Morbidity and Mortality Weekly Report. 68(3): 1-32.
33. Health Service Executive (HSE). (2009). Use of personal protective equipment (PPE) in healthcare settings.
34. Yunus, M.B., and Mense, S. (2019). Myofascial pain syndrome and trigger points: clinical review and pathophysiology. Pain Medicine. 21(2): 179-190.
35. Cagnie, B., Dewitte, V., Barbe, T., Timmermans, F., Delrue, N. (2020). Needling therapies in the management of myofascial trigger points: A systematic review. American Journal of Physical Medicine and Rehabilitation. 99(4): 309-318.
36. Gattie, E., Cleland, J.A., Snodgrass, S.J. (2017). Dry needling for patients with musculoskeletal pain: A clinical commentary. International Journal of Sports Physical Therapy. 12(2): 227-236.
37. Kietrys, D. M., Palombaro, K. M., Azzaretto, E. (2019). Effectiveness of dry needling for upper-quarter myofascial pain: A systematic review and meta-analysis. Journal of Orthopaedic and Sports Physical Therapy. 43(9): 620-634.
38. Shah, J. P., Thaker, N. (2018). Myofascial pain and nociceptive trigger points: Time to integrate dry needling with evidence-based medicine. The Journal of Orthopaedic and Sports Physical Therapy. 48(1): 3-9.

39. Melzack, R., Wall, P.D. (1965). Pain mechanisms: a new theory. Science, 150(3699): 971-979.
40. Dommerholt, J., Fernández-de-las-Peñas, C. (2013). Trigger Point Dry Needling: An Evidence and Clinical-Based Approach. Churchill Livingstone.
41. Shah, J.P., Gilliams, E.A. (2008). Uncovering the biochemical milieu of myofascial trigger points using in vivo microdialysis: An application of muscle pain concepts to myofascial pain syndrome. Journal of Bodywork and Movement Therapies. 12(4): 371-384.
42. Langevin, H.M., Yandow, J.A. (2002). Relationship of acupuncture points and meridians to connective tissue planes. The Anatomical Record. 269(6): 257-265.
43. Hidalgo, J., Torres, M., Mayoral, O., Sanchez, Z., Prieto, S. (2013). Infrared thermography for the detection of myofascial trigger points in patients with neck pain. Medical Physics. 40(7).
44. Dutton, M. (2018). Fundamentals of Musculoskeletal Assessment Techniques. 4th ed. New York: Elsevier.
45. Kettner, N., Ragnarsdottir, M. (2014). The Importance of Medical History and Physical Examination in the Clinical Setting. Journal of Physical Therapy Science. 26(4): 649-653.
46. Gillon, R. (2015). Informed Consent: A Guide for Healthcare Professionals. Journal of Medical Ethics. 41(5): 391-395.
47. Riazi, H., Dyer, C. B. (2016). Informed Consent: Ethical and Legal Considerations in Physical Therapy Practice. Physiotherapy Theory and Practice. 32(1): 37-46.
48. Groves, M. (2016). Documenting Informed Consent in Physical Therapy: An Ethical and Legal Imperative. Journal of Physical Therapy Education. 30(3): 15-22.
49. Schenck, K.L., Hall, R.M. (2018). Legal Considerations in Informed Consent for Physical Therapy. Journal of Legal Medicine. 39(3): 331-344.
50. McEwen, I.R., Pomeranz, B. (2015). Clinical Handbook of Physiotherapy. New York: Wiley.
51. Walker, J.A., Allen, S.S. (2017). Infection Control in Physical Therapy Practice. Journal of Physical Therapy Science. 29(9): 1665-1670.
52. Glover, J.E., Pomeranz, B. (2016). Patient Positioning and Ergonomics in Rehabilitation. Physical Therapy. 96(5): 617-626.

53. Sweeney, J., Murphy, A. (2019). Best Practices for Patient Positioning in Manual Therapy Techniques. Physiotherapy Theory and Practice. 35(2): 136-142.
54. Cummings, T.M., Cummings, T.J. (2015). Dry Needling: A Clinical Perspective. Journal of Manual and Manipulative Therapy. 23(3): 145-155.
55. Dommerholt, J. (2011). Myofascial Trigger Points: Pathophysiology and Evidence-Informed Diagnosis and Management. Journal of Manual and Manipulative Therapy. 19(3): 137-147.
56. Trevelyan, F.C., and Noyes, R.A. (2018). Post-Needling Care: Understanding the Role of Patient Education. Physical Therapy Reviews. 23(1): 22-31.
57. Alvarez, A. (2015). Dry needling: efficacy in the treatment of myofascial pain syndrome. International Journal of Medicine and Sciences of Physical Activity and Sport. 15(59): 245-258.
58. Sato, T., Rosen, J. (2020). Effects of dry needling on muscle pain: a systematic review. Physiotherapy Theory and Practice. 36(4): 428-441.
59. Ursini, T., Tontodonati, M. (2018). The role of inflammation in muscle regeneration. Current Opinion in Rheumatology. 30(1): 38-43.
60. Shah, J.P., Thaker, H. (2023). "Nonmyofascial Trigger Points: A Comprehensive Review." Journal of Pain Research. 16: 107-119.
61. Klein, M.J., et al. (2021). "Non-myo-fascial Trigger Points: An Underrecognized Cause of Pain." Journal of Bodywork and Movement Therapies. 25(4): 767-773.
62. Alvarez, D. J., Rockwell, P. G. (2022). "Understanding Non-Myo-Fascial Pain: A Review of Trigger Points and Related Conditions." Pain Medicine. 23(8): 1433-1442.
63. Meyer, M.F., et al. (2022). "Exploring the Mechanisms Behind Dry Needling in Non-myofascial Pain: An Evidence-Based Approach." Clinical Rehabilitation. 36(6): 760-771.
64. Tashjian, R.Z., et al. (2021). "Clinical Approaches to Nonmyofascial Trigger Points." Pain Physician. 24(2): 97-106.
65. Tough, E.A., White, A.R. (2022). "The Role of Dry Needling in Treating Non-Myo-fascial Pain." Current Pain and Headache Reports. 26(6): 455-462.
66. Mayoral, O., Salvat, I. (2021). Invasive physiotherapy of myofascial pain syndrome: trigger point dry needling manual. ISBN: 978-8491103950.

67. Alonso, C., Fernández, C. (2010). Is dry needling effective in the management of myofascial trigger points associated with neck pain? Clinical Journal of Pain. 26(3): 284-292.
68. Gonzalez, L.M., Infante, P., Granados, M., Urresti, F.J. (2015). Myofascial pain syndrome associated with the temporomandibular joint: a review of current management. Journal of Oral and Maxillofacial Surgery. 73(1): 141-147.
69. Jaeger, B., Reeves, J.L. (2009). Myofascial Trigger Point Pathophysiology: Current Concepts. PM&R. 1(2): 180-194.
70. Fernández, C., Cuadrado, M.L. (2014). Myofascial headaches: pathophysiology and management strategies. Expert Review of Neurotherapeutics. 14(3): 311-322.
71. Chou, M., Widmer, C.G. (2010). Management of Myofascial Pain of the Jaw Muscles: A Review. Journal of the American Dental Association. 141(4): 459-467.
72. Gerwin, R. D. (2001). Classification, Epidemiology, and Natural History of Myofascial Pain Syndrome. Current Pain and Headache Reports. 5(5): 412-420.
73. Okeson, J.P. (2013). Management of Temporomandibular Disorders and Occlusion. Elsevier Health Sciences.
74. Stecco, C. (2014). Functional Atlas of the Human Fascial System. Elsevier Health Sciences.
75. Fernandez, C., & Arendt, L. (2016). Myofascial Trigger Points: Comprehensive Diagnosis and Treatment. Springer.
76. Hanten, W.P., Olson, S.L., Russell, J.L., Lucio, R.M. (2000). "Effectiveness of a Home Program of Ischemic Pressure Followed by Sustained Stretch for Treatment of Myofascial Trigger Points." Physical Therapy. 80(10): 997-1003.
77. Fernandez, C., Dommerholt, J. (2018). Clinical Guide to Musculoskeletal Palpation: A Practical Guide. Elsevier.
78. Bron, C., de Gast, A., Dommerholt, J., Stegenga, B. (2011). "Trigger Points and Central Sensitization in Musculoskeletal Pain Disorders." Pain Medicine. 12(3): 328-333.
79. Bron, C., Dommerholt, J. (2012). "Dry Needling of Myofascial Trigger Points in the Scalene Muscles." Journal of Manual & Manipulative Therapy. 20(4): 208-216.
80. Lewis, J., Tehan, P. (2010). "Thoracic Outlet Syndrome and the Role of Myofascial Trigger Points." Physical Therapy Reviews. 15(2): 135-145.

81. Moseley, G.L., Butler, D.S. (2015). Focal Brain Changes in Chronic Pain: A Review. Neuroscience and Biobehavioral Reviews. 52: 94-104.
82. Cameron, M.H., Monroe, L.G. (2011). "Rehabilitation of the Spine: A Patient-Centered Approach." Journal of Orthopaedic and Sports Physical Therapy. 41(4): 252-259.
83. Elvey, R. (2009). "The Role of the Cervical Musculature in Cervicogenic Headaches." Physiotherapy Theory and Practice. 25(3): 167-179.
84. Kothari, M. J., Zhang, C. (2020). "Cervical Muscles: Function and Dysfunction." Physical Therapy Reviews. 25(1): 4-10.
85. Fernández-de-Las-Peñas, C., & Cuadrado, M.L. (2007). "Tension-Type Headache and Myofascial Trigger Points: A Review of the Literature". Current Pain and Headache Reports. 11(6): 465-472.
86. Hallgren, R.C., Greenman, P.E., Rechtien, J.J. (1994). "Chronic Cervical Pain and Headache: Postural Considerations". Journal of Manipulative and Physiological Therapeutics. 17(6): 375-379.
87. Lopez, C., et al. (2013). "Immediate Effects of Active Stretching on Pain and Pressure Pain Sensitivity Over Myofascial Trigger Points in the Upper Trapezius and Levator Scapulae: A Randomized Controlled Trial". Journal of Manipulative and Physiological Therapeutics. 36(6): 379-387.
88. Chaitow, L., DeLany, J.W. (2011). Clinical Application of Neuromuscular Techniques, Volume 1: The Upper Body (2nd Ed.). Churchill Livingstone.
89. Bron, C., et al. (2011). "Prevalence of Myofascial Trigger Points in Patients with Chronic Shoulder Pain". Journal of Manual & Manipulative Therapy. 19(1): 11-17.
90. Fernandez, C., Cleland, J.A., Huijbregts, P. (2015). Manual Therapy for Musculoskeletal Pain Syndromes: An Evidence and Clinical Informed Approach. Elsevier.
91. Shah, J.P., Gilliams, E.A. (2008). "Uncovering the Biochemical Milieu of Myofascial Trigger Points Using in Vivo Microdialysis: An Application of Muscle Pain Concepts to Myofascial Pain Syndrome." Journal of Bodywork and Movement Therapies. 12(4): 371-384.
92. Fernandez, C., Simons, D., Cuadrado, M.L., Gerwin, R.D. (2015). Trigger Points and Muscle Chains in Osteopathy. Elsevier.
93. Gatts, S., Currier, L., Baker, R. (2021). "Anatomical, Functional, and Myofascial Insights Into the Teres Minor: Implications for Shoulder Rehabilitation." Journal of Rehabilitation Research and Practice.

94. De la Llave, A.I., Fernandez, J., Ortega, R. (2020). "Dry Needling in Myofascial Pain Syndrome: Update and Future Directions." Current Pain and Headache Reports. 24(2): 9.
95. Salamh, P.A., Lewis, J.S. (2021). "Myofascial Trigger Points: An Evidence-Informed Review." Journal of Manual & Manipulative Therapy. 29(3): 147-154.
96. Liu, L., Huang, Q.M., Liu, Q.G., Ye, G., Bo, C.Z., Chen, M.J., Li, P. (2015). Effectiveness of dry needling for myofascial trigger points associated with neck and shoulder pain: a systematic review and meta-analysis. Arch Phys Med Rehabil. 96(5):944-55.
97. Kumar, A., Gupta, K. (2016). Puncture Dry Needling in Myofascial Pain Syndromes: An Overview. International Journal of Clinical Rheumatology. 11(3): 179-189.
98. Hopper, D.J. (2008). The Role of the Latissimus Dorsi Muscle in Shoulder Function: A Biomechanical Review. Journal of Orthopaedic & Sports Physical Therapy, 38(4), 252-258.
99. Hassan, M., Khedher, I. (2021). Management of Myofascial Pain Syndrome: A Review of the Evidence. European Journal of Physical and Rehabilitation Medicine. 57(3): 365-375.
100. Hwang, S.Y., et al. (2015). The Effectiveness of Dry Needling for Myofascial Trigger Points in Musculoskeletal Disorders: A Systematic Review and Meta-Analysis. Physical Therapy. 95(11): 1545-1558.
101. Kumar, V., & Clark, M.L. (2020). Clinical Medicine. Elsevier. ISBN: 9780702078682
102. Urits, I., Charipova, K., Gress, K., Schaaf, A.L., Gupta, S., Kiernan, H.C., et al. (2020). Treatment and management of myofascial pain syndrome. Best Pract Res Clin Anaesthesiol. 34(3):427-448.
103. Ong, J., Claydon, L.S. (2014). The effect of dry needling for myofascial trigger points in the neck and shoulders: a systematic review and meta-analysis. J Bodyw Mov Ther. 18(3): 390-8.
104. Liu, L, Huang, Q.M., Liu, Q.G., Ye, G., Bo, C.Z., Chen, M.J., et al. (2015). Effectiveness of dry needling for myofascial trigger points associated with neck and shoulder pain: a systematic review and meta-analysis. Arch Phys Med Rehabil. 96(5): 944-55.
105. Chys, M., De Meulemeester, K., De Greef, I., Murillo, C., Kindt, W., Kouzouz, Y., et al. (2023). Clinical Effectiveness of Dry Needling in Patients with Musculoskeletal Pain-An Umbrella Review. J Clin Med. 12(3):1205.

106. Dunning, J., Butts, R., Mourad, F., Young, I., Flannagan, S., Perreault, T. (2014). Dry needling: a literature review with implications for clinical practice guidelines. Phys Ther Rev. 19(4):252-265.
107. Borg, J., Iaccarino, M.A. (2014). Myofascial pain syndrome treatments. Phys Med Rehabil Clin N Am. 25(2):357-74.
108. Wendt, M., Waszak, M. (2020). Evaluation of the Combination of Muscle Energy Technique and Trigger Point Therapy in Asymptomatic Individuals with a Latent Trigger Point. Int J Environ Res Public Health. 17(22):8430.
109. Mense, S. (2008). Muscle pain: mechanisms and clinical significance. 105(12): 214-9.
110. Espejo, L., Fernández, J., Albornoz, M., Rodríguez, J., De la Cruz, B., Ribeiro, F., Silva, A. (2017). Dry needling in the management of myofascial trigger points: A systematic review of randomized controlled trials. 33: 46-57.
111. Ma, Y.T., Ma, M. (2011). Biomedical Acupuncture for Sports and Trauma Rehabilitation: Dry Needling Techniques. Elsevier Health Sciences.
112. Navarro, M.J., Sanchez, J., Gómez, G.F., Cleland, J.A., López, I., Fernández, C., et al. (2020). Effects of trigger point dry needling on lateral epicondylalgia of musculoskeletal origin: A systematic review and meta-analysis. Clinical Rehabilitation. 34: 1327-1340.
113. Kalichman L, Vulfsons S (2010). Dry needling in the management of musculoskeletal pain. Journal of the American Board of Family Medicine. 23:640-646.
114. Dommerholt J., Fernandez, C., Petersen, S.M. (2019). Needling: Is there a point?. Journal of Manual and Manipulative Therapy. 27 :125-127.
115. Cagnie, B., Dewitte, V., Barbe, T., Timmermans, F., Delrue, N., Meeus, M. (2013). Physiologic effects of dry needling. Current Pain and Headache Reports. 17:348.
116. Charles, D., Hudgins, T., MacNaughton, J., Newman, E., Tan, J., Wigger, M. (2019). A systematic review of manual therapy techniques, dry cupping and dry needling in the reduction of myofascial pain and myofascial trigger points. Journal of Bodywork and Movement Therapies. 23: 539-546.
117. Rodríguez, J., González, B., De Toro, Á., Valera, E., Garrido, E.M., Jiménez, M. (2016). Effectiveness of dry needling on reducing pain

intensity in patients with myofascial pain syndrome: A Meta-analysis. Journal of Traditional Chinese Medicine. 36: 1-13.

118. Sánchez, J., Navarro, M.J., Bravo, A., Jiménez, F., Abián, J. (2021). Is Dry Needling Applied by Physical Therapists Effective for Pain in Musculoskeletal Conditions? A Systematic Review and Meta-Analysis. Physical Therapy. 101(3).

119. Tough, E.A., White, A.R., Cummings, T.M., Richards, S.H., Campbell, J.L. (2009). Acupuncture and dry needling in the management of myofascial trigger point pain: A systematic review and meta-analysis of randomised controlled trials. European Journal of Pain. 13: 3-10.

120. Dommerholt, J. (2011). Dry needling Peripheral and central considerations. Journal of Manual & Manipulative Therapy. 19: 223-227.

121. Hall, M.L., Mackie, A.C., Ribeiro, D.C. (2018). Effects of dry needling trigger point therapy in the shoulder region on patients with upper extremity pain and dysfunction: A systematic review with meta-analysis. Physiotherapy. 104: 167-177.

122. Boyles, R., Fowler, R., Ramsey, D., Burrows, E. (2015). Effectiveness of trigger point dry needling for multiple body regions: A systematic review. Journal of Manual & Manipulative Therapy. 23: 276-293.

123. Lew, J., Kim, J., Nair, P. (2021). Comparison of dry needling and trigger point manual therapy in patients with neck and upper back myofascial pain syndrome: A systematic review and meta-analysis. Journal of Manual & Manipulative Therapy. 29: 136-146.

124. Fernandez, C., Nijs, J. (2019). Trigger point dry needling for the treatment of myofascial pain syndrome: Current perspectives within a pain neuroscience paradigm. Pain Management Journal. 12: 1899-1911.

125. Butts, R., Dunning, J., Serafino, C. (2021). Dry needling strategies for musculoskeletal conditions: Do the number of needles and needle retention time matter? A narrative literature review. Journal of Bodywork and Movement Therapies. 26: 353-363.

126. Uygur, E., Aktas, B., Özkut, A., et al. (2017). Dry needling in lateral epicondylitis: a prospective controlled study. Int Orthop. 41(11): 2321-2325.

127. Kheradmandi, A., Ebrahimian, M., Ghafarinejad, F., et al. (2015). The effect of dry needling of the trigger points of shoulder muscles on

pain and grip strength in patients with lateral epicondylitis: a pilot study. J Rehabil Sci Res. 2(3): 58-62.

128. Sukumar, S., Sukumar, S., Lawrence, M.S. (2014). Effects of static dry needle insertion and trigger point deactivation combined with eccentric exercises in women with unilateral tennis elbow, a single blinded RCT. Glob J Multidiscip Stud. 4(1): 411-422.

129. Ukumar, S., Lawrence, M., Subhashchandra, R. (2015). Early effects of dry needling and low-level laser therapy in chronic tennis elbow: an experimental study. J Heal Sci Res. 5(1): 187-196.

130. Etminan, Z., Razeghi, M., Ghafarinejad, F. (2019). The effect of dry needling of trigger points in forearm's extensor muscles on the grip force, pain and function of athletes with chronic tennis elbow. J Rehabil Sci Res. 6(1): 27-33.

131. Tekin, L., Akarsu, S., Durmus, O., Cakar, E., Dincer, U., Kiralp, M.Z. (2013). The effect of dry needling in the treatment of myofascial pain syndrome: a randomized double-blinded placebo-controlled trial. Clin Rheumatol. 32(3): 309-15.

132. Hsieh, Y.L., Kao, M.J., Kuan, T.S., Chen, S.M., Chen, J.T., Hong, C.Z. (2007). Dry needling to a key myofascial trigger point may reduce the irritability of satellite MTrPs. Am J Phys Med Rehabil. 86(5): 397-403.

133. Irnich, D., Behrens, J., Gleditsch, J.M., et al. (2002). Immediate effects of dry needling and acupuncture at distant points in chronic neck pain: results of a randomized, double-blind, sham-controlled crossover trial. 99(1-2): 83-89

134. Lorenzo, L., Traballesi, M., Morelli, D., et al. (2004). Hemiparetic Shoulder Pain Syndrome Treated with Deep Dry Needling During Early Rehabilitation: A Prospective, Open-Label, Randomized Investigation. J Musculoskelet Pain. 12(2): 25-34

135. Tsai, C.T., Hsieh, L.F., Kuan, T.S. (2010). Remote effects of dry needling on the irritability of the myofascial trigger point in the upper trapezius muscle. Am J Phys Med Rehabil. 89(2): 133-140.

136. García, R., Tormos, L., Vilanova, P., Morales, R., Pérez, A., Segura, E. (2011). Effectiveness of dry needling of a myofascial trigger point versus elbow manipulation on pain and maximal hand grip strength. Physiotherapy. 33(6): 248-255.

137. Mansfield, C.J., Vanetten, L., Willy, R., Magnussen, R., Briggs, M. (2019). The effects of needling therapies on muscle force production:

A systematic review and meta-analysis. Journal of Orthopaedic and Sports Physical Therapy.

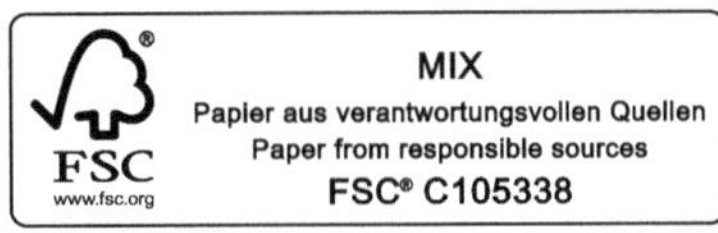

Printed by Books on Demand GmbH, Norderstedt / Germany